NEW PERSPECTIVES IN BREAST IMAGING

Edited by **Arshad M. Malik**

New Perspectives in Breast Imaging
http://dx.doi.org/10.5772/67606
Edited by Arshad M. Malik

Contributors

Ryusuke Murakami, Nachiko Uchiyama, Hitomi Tani, Shinichiro Kumita, Jose Maria Celaya-Padilla, Jorge Issac Galvan-Tejada, Carlos Eric Galvan-Tejada, Cesar Humberto Guzman-Valdivia, Hamurabi Gamboa Rosales, Juan Ruben Delgado-Contreras, Victor Trevino, Jose Gerardo Tamez-Peña, Jorge Roberto Manjarrez Sánchez, Antonio Martinez-Torteya, Roberto Olivera Reyna, Francisco Javier Martinez Ruiz, Idalia Garza-Veloz, Margarita Martinez-Fierro, Shinya Tajima, Yoshihiko Kuwahara, Geetha Manjunath, Siva Teja Kakileti, Himanshu Madhu, Ramprakash Hv, Alexander Karpov, Ashkan Ghanbarzadeh Dagheyan, Jose Angel Martinez Lorenzo, Lulu Wang, Hu Peng, Jianhua Ma, Mohammed Ali Alnafea

Published by InTech
Janeza Trdine 9, 51000 Rijeka, Croatia

Publishing Process Manager Nina Kalinic
Technical Editor SPi Global
Cover InTech Design team

First published September, 2017
Printed in Croatia
Legal deposit, Croatia: National and University Library in Zagreb

Additional hard copies can be obtained from orders@intechopen.com

New Perspectives in Breast Imaging, Edited by Arshad M. Malik
p. cm.
Print ISBN 978-953-51-3557-9
Online ISBN 978-953-51-3558-6

For EU product safety concerns:
IN TECH d.o.o., Prolaz Marije Krucifikse Kozulić 3, 51000 Rijeka, Croatia,
info@intechopen.com or visit our website at intechopen.com.

Meet the editor

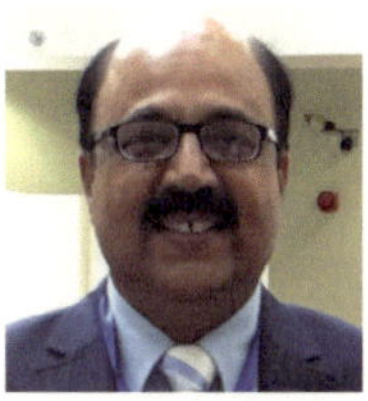

Dr. Arshad Malik is a graduate of Liaquat University of Medical and Health Sciences wherein he completed his training in surgery under supervision of Professor Jan Mohammad Memon (FRCS).

He is presently working as associate professor of Surgery at College of Medicine, Qassim University, Saudi Arabia. He is a reviewer of many international journals. He is the author of 49 national and international scientific papers that are well appreciated in the health community. Dr. Malik has presented his work in many international and national conferences. He has attended many workshops and seminars all over the world. He is an editor of two books on laparoscopic surgery. He has also contributed chapters in books that have attracted a huge readership.

Contents

Preface

Breast cancer is the most widely recognized obtrusive disease in females and the second in number among lethal cancers, after lung tumor. Early detection of this cancer can have a very good prognosis and quality of life. As the familiarity with the malignancy has become rife among ladies, increasing use of screening programs has turned out to be broadly acknowledged as a vital piece of women health. It is a well-established fact that an early recognition of disease or precancerous lesions can diminish morbidity and mortality, mental health, and financial trauma to the individual and society. There is a global concern now in providing superb screening and analytic facilities to ladies who are underserved and do not have an easy access to such facilities. A number of modalities to diagnose this cancer are in practice. Mammography is the most common tool for this purpose but has a low sensitivity. On the other hand, the utilization of ultrasound for breast tumor screening acquires a high rate of false-negative outcomes, especially in ladies with dense breast tissue. Therefore, Ultrasound is by and large utilized as a supplement to mammography amid screening to enhance identification, particularly for ladies with dense breasts.

This book is focused to the latest radiological concepts to make it possible to save more and more lives by way of early detection and treatment of the cancer while it is at its very early stages. There are many high-quality contributions from most eminent scientists all around. I hope this book will benefit both the practicing surgeons and residents of surgery and radiology and will definitely bring a phenomenal change in the outlook of breast cancer patients.

Dr. Arshad M. Malik
College of Medicine, Department of Surgery
Qassim University, Saudi Arabia

Chapter 1

A Case of an Invasive Lobular Carcinoma with Extracellular Mucin: Radio-Pathological Correlation

Shinya Tajima, Keiko Kishimoto,
Yoshihide Kanemaki, Ichiro Maeda, Akira Endo,
Motohiro Chosokabe, Takafumi Ono,
Koichiro Tsugawa and Masayuki Takagi

Additional information is available at the end of the chapter

http://dx.doi.org/10.5772/intechopen.69389

Abstract

A case of 77-year-old female with an invasive lobular carcinoma with extracellular mucin is presented. She felt palpable mass in her left breast. Then, she came to our hospital for further examination. Mammography of right in full view revealed architectural distortion in left upper portion. And ultrasonography demonstrated low-echoic mass about 2 cm in diameter and invasion of the fat tissue was observed. Hence, malignancy was suspected and magnetic resonance imaging (MRI) was performed. MRI findings showed irregular shaped and margined mass with small T2-high-signal intensity. These findings suggested invasive carcinoma with mucin. Because the cancer lesion was not large, partial mastectomy was performed. Interestingly, pathological diagnosis was invasive lobular carcinoma with extracellular mucin. Extracellular mucinous lesion was concordant with small T2-high-signal intensity. This type of carcinoma was previously reported only in three cases, and rare but important, because the treatment and prognosis might change by histological subtypes. We suggest one of the MRI special features of our case is not only irregular shaped and margined mass but also small T2-high-signal intensity. These MR findings might be one of the valuable findings for the diagnosis and differentiation between this type of carcinoma from other tumors.

Keywords: magnetic resonance imaging, breast, invasive lobular carcinoma, extracellular mucin, E-cadherin

1. Introduction

To discriminate between invasive lobular carcinoma and invasive ductal carcinoma is a big theme for both radiologically and pathologically. The limitation of radiologic imaging in the detection and evaluation of invasive lobular carcinoma have been recognized for a long time. Whereas, advances in breast radiologic imaging present opportunities to improve the diagnosis of invasive lobular carcinoma.

On mammography, invasive lobular carcinoma is not likely to form calcifications. However, calcifications may be present in benign proliferative lesions such as sclerosing adenosis [1]. The most common manifestations of invasive lobular carcinoma are asymmetric density, irregular, or spiculated mass on mammography [2–4].

On ultrasonography, 60.5% of invasive lobular carcinomas produced "a heterogeneous low-echoic mass with angular or irregular margins and posterior acoustic shadowing." The remaining tumors had various other sonographic characteristics, including 12% that were "ultrasonographically invisible." The sensitivity of ultrasonography for tumors measuring less than 1 cm was 85.7%. Invasive lobular carcinoma of common type tended to produce "focal shadowing without a discrete mass," whereas tumors with pleomorphic histology were seen as "a shadowing mass." Tumors of the alveolar, solid, and signet-ring variant of invasive lobular carcinoma were most often manifested as a "lobulated, well circumscribed mass" [5]. Ultrasonography is useful and more accurate than mammography in diagnosing invasive lobular carcinoma [5]. However, it is difficult to narrow down the diagnosis of invasive lobular carcinoma.

Breast magnetic resonance imaging (MRI) has an overall sensitivity of 93% for detecting invasive lobular carcinoma, similar to the detection of breast cancers overall (90%). On MRI, tumor of smooth margin, or absence of smooth margin and the distribution of nonmass-like enhancement are the features of invasive lobular carcinoma. Invasive lobular carcinoma may present as ductal, segmental, regional, or diffuse patterns [6]. MR imaging is considered to be a useful tool for detecting invasive lobular carcinoma on radiologically.

Pathologically, the invasive lobular carcinoma includes not only classical type (Foote and Stewart advocated in 1946 [7]) but also variants of solid, alveolar, pleomorphic, tubulolobular, signet-ring, trabecular, and mixed types [8].

We encountered a tumor of invasive carcinoma coexisting with mucinous carcinoma-like lesion. At first, the differential diagnoses of this tumor are (i) mixed mucinous-ductal carcinoma, (ii) mucinous carcinoma with neuroendocrine feature, (iii) mucinous papillary neoplasms, and (iv) carcinoma of mixed type (lobular and ductal carcinoma). Lobular carcinoma has been considered a variant of mucin-secreting carcinoma with only intracytoplasmic mucin [9–11]. In common practice, a diagnosis of mucinous carcinoma or ductal carcinoma with mucinous features is often made in the presence of extracellular mucin, without immunohistochemical confirmation of the ductal phenotype [10]. However, final diagnosis was "invasive lobular carcinoma with extracellular mucin" which has been reported only in three cases in the English medical literature [9–11]. Accordingly, the current report is the fourth documented case in pathology, and in the viewpoint of radiology, this is the first case.

Taking into consideration of the above information, we will discuss the unique variant of "invasive lobular carcinoma with extracellular mucin" with radiopathological correlation.

2. Materials and methods

2.1. MR imaging protocol

MR imaging was performed using a 1.5T MR system (Achieva 1.5T, Philips Healthcare Nederland, Eindhoven, Netherland), and a synergy breast coil. Routine breast MR images were acquired as follows in the prone position: axial T2-weighted turbo spin echo (TSE) with STIR images (repetition time (TR)/echo time (TE) = 5175/60 ms, section thickness = 5 mm, FOV = 280 mm, matrix = 480 × 480), and axial diffusion-weighted (DW) images using a single-shot EPI (FOV = 280 mm, matrix = 128 × 128), with MPG pulse applied along three directions (x, y, and z axes) with TR/TE of 5532/80 ms and b-factors of 0, 1000, and 2000 s/mm^2. Apparent diffusion coefficient (ADC)-maps were automatically generated on a postprocessing workstation. After axial T1-weighted SE images, [TR/TE = 468.8/12 ms, flip angle = 90, section thickness = 5 mm, FOV = 280 mm, matrix = 128 × 128] were obtained, axial 3D dynamic contrast enhanced T1-weighted images with SPAIR using eTHRIVE sequence [TR/TE = 5.9/2.8 ms, flip angle = 10, section thickness = 5 mm, FOV = 280 mm, matrix = 512 × 512] were performed in precontrast, double arterial phase, and delayed phase.

2.2. Image interpretation

For image interpretation of mammography, ultrasonography, and magnetic resonance imaging, we used the breast imaging and reporting data system (BI-RADS) lexicon and associated report of Tozaki et al. [12, 13].

2.3. Hematoxylin and eosin staining

Operation samples obtained from the partial mastectomy were fixed at least 8 h in 10% neutral phosphate buffered formalin, then, embedded in paraffin, and sectioned at 3–4 μm. The paraffin-embedded specimens were stained with hematoxylin and eosin (HE) for light microscopic examination.

2.4. Immunohistochemistry

Paraffin-embedded sections measuring 3–4 μm thick were deparaffinized. Antigen retrieval was then performed for 20–40 min in boiling water (95°C) containing citric acid solution (pH 6.0) or Target Retrieval Solution (pH 9.0; cat. no. 415211; Nichirei, Tokyo, Japan), and (pH 6.0; cat. no. S2031; Dako, Glostrup, Denmark). Sections were pretreated with 0.3% peroxide and reacted with primary monoclonal antibodies against estrogen receptor (ER), progesterone receptor (PgR), HER2, Ki67, E-cadherin, Synaptophysin, MUC1, and MUC3 are shown in **Table 1**. Subsequently, specimens were incubated with a secondary antibody (Histofine simple stain MAX-PO; cat. no. 424154; Nichirei). The chromogenic substrate was 3,3′-diaminobenzidine (DAB), and the slides were counterstained with hematoxylin.

Antibody	Clone	Source	Activation	Dilution
ER	EP1	DAKO	Heat pH 9.0/40 min	1:2
PgR	PgR636	DAKO	Heat pH 6.0/40 min	1:2
HER2	Rabbit poly	DAKO	Heat pH 6.0/40 min	1:1
Ki-67	MIB-1	DAKO	Heat pH 6.0/40 min	1:200
E-cadherin	35B5	Leica	Heat pH 6.0/40 min	1:2
Synaptophysin	27G12	NICHIREI	Heat pH 9.0/40 min	1:2
MUC1	Ma552	Leica	Heat pH 6.0/40 min	1:100
MUC3	1143/B7	Lab Vision	Heat pH 6.0/40 min	1:100

Table 1. Primary monoclonal antibodies against ER, PgR, HER2, Ki67, E-cadherin, synaptophysin, MUC1, and MUC3.

3. Results

A case of 77-year-old female is presented. She felt palpable mass in her left breast since 1 month and came to our hospital for further examination.

Physical examination revealed a 2.7 cm palpable mass in left upper inner and outer quadrants without nipple discharge and lymphadenopathy. No familial history of breast cancer was confirmed.

On mammography, the breast appeared dense. However, mediolateral oblique (MLO) view of the mammography demonstrated architectural distortion in left upper portion (**Figure 1**). Hence, this lesion was of four categories. Right MLO view revealed no evidence of malignancy.

Ultrasonography revealed a low-echoic mass about 2 cm in diameter with posterior acoustic shadowing, and disruption of the anterior border line (the anterior border line means boundary line between fat tissue layer and breast parenchymal layer) of the mass was observed in her left breast (**Figure 2**). There was no lesion suggesting malignancy in her right breast. No lymph node swelling was seen.

These findings suggested the possibility of malignancy. Therefore, magnetic resonance imaging (MRI) of 1.5T (Philips) was performed. On MRI, diffusion-weighted image of b-value 1000 s/mm^2 showed mass-like lesion with high signal intensity (**Figure 3A**). Apparent diffusion coefficient (ADC)-map revealed diffusion limitation of the water molecule (**Figure 3B**). Dynamic contrast-enhanced T1 weighted images demonstrated early enhancement and delayed washout pattern of irregular shaped and margined mass about

http://dx.doi.org/10.5772/intechopen.69389

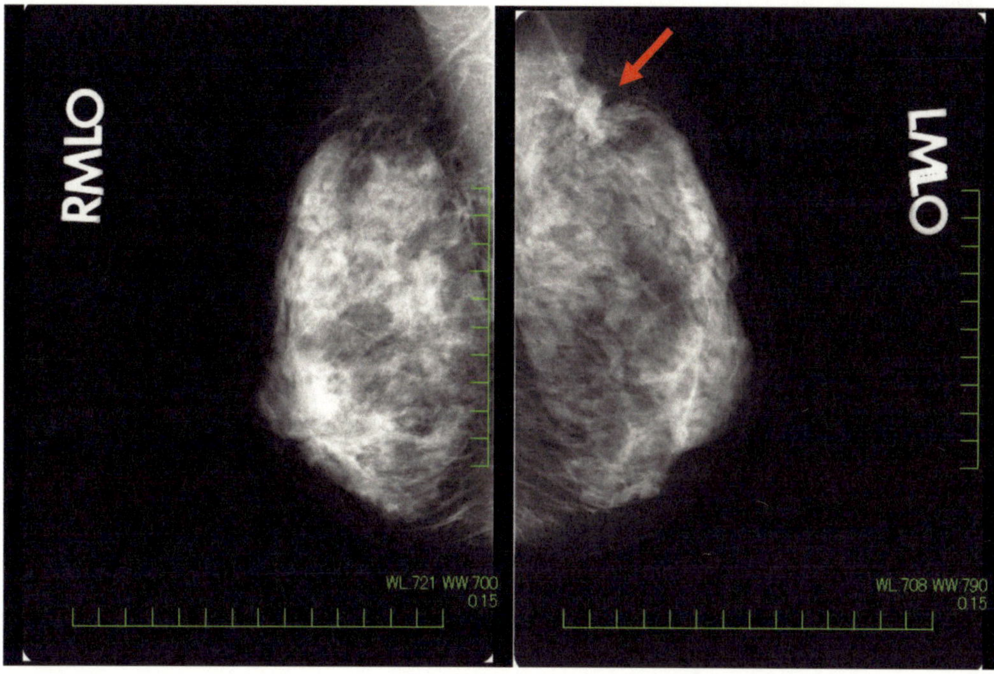

Figure 1. MLO view of the mammography demonstrates architectural distortion in left upper portion (arrow).

2 cm in diameter (**Figure 3C** and **D**). The mass included a small high signal intensity area on fat-saturated T2 weighted image, which was confirmed pathologically as extracellular mucin. (**Figure 3E**). Dynamic-curve of the contrast-enhanced MRI showed rapid wash-out pattern (**Figure 3F**). ADC value was 0.577×10^{-3} mm^2/s; hence, the existence of water restriction was suggested.

Neoadjuvant chemotherapy was not performed. Then, partial mastectomy was performed because of the imaging findings. Sentinel lymph node was negative for metastatic cancer lesion. Further, axillary lymph node resection was not performed. Histopathological findings revealed low-grade tumor with little or no nuclear atypia and inconspicuous nucleoli. Besides, the tumor was composed of single cell with moderate pleomorphism and lack of cohesion. The neoplastic cells were arranged in files or cords infiltrating the stroma. Partially, trabecular type lesion was observed (**Figure 4A**). Within the tumor, there were areas showing signet-ring cells floating in a pool of mucin (**Figure 4B**). The presence of the extracellular mucin is not a characteristic of lobular carcinomas. Therefore, immunohistochemical stain for E-cadherin was performed. However, the lesions were negative for E-cadherin immunostaining (**Figure 4C**). Besides, neuroendocrine marker of synaptophysin was completely negative. MIB1 (Ki67)-index was about 10%. Estrogen receptor (ER), progesterone receptor (PgR), and human epidermal growth factor receptor 2 (HER2) status were 99, 0%, and negative, respectively. Additionally, special stainings for mucin as MUC1 and MUC3 were performed, and both stainings were positive of both infiltrating cells and signet-ring cells floating in a pool of mucin (**Figure 4D** and **E**).

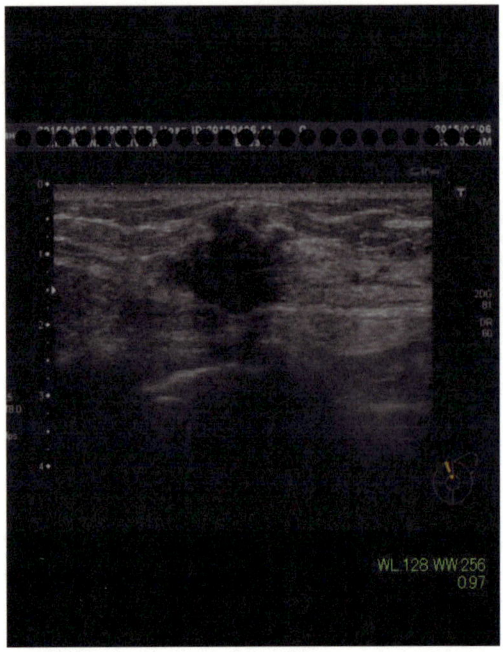

Figure 2. Ultrasonography reveals a low-echoic mass, posterior acoustic shadowing, and disruption of the anterior border line is observed.

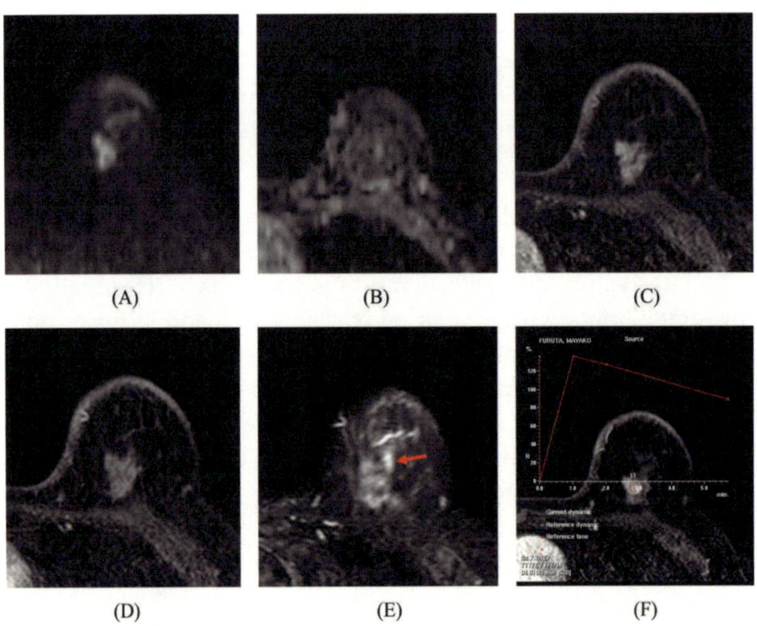

Figure 3. (A) Diffusion-weighted image of b-1000 shows mass like high signal intensity. (B) Apparent diffusion coefficient (ADC)-map reveals diffusion limitation of the water molecule. (C) Contrast-enhanced T1 weighted images demonstrate early enhancement and (D) delayed washout pattern. (E) The mass included a small high-signal intensity on fat-saturated T2 weighted image, which is confirmed pathologically as extracellular mucin (arrow). (F) Dynamic-curve of the MRI shows rapid washout pattern.

http://dx.doi.org/10.5772/intechopen.69389

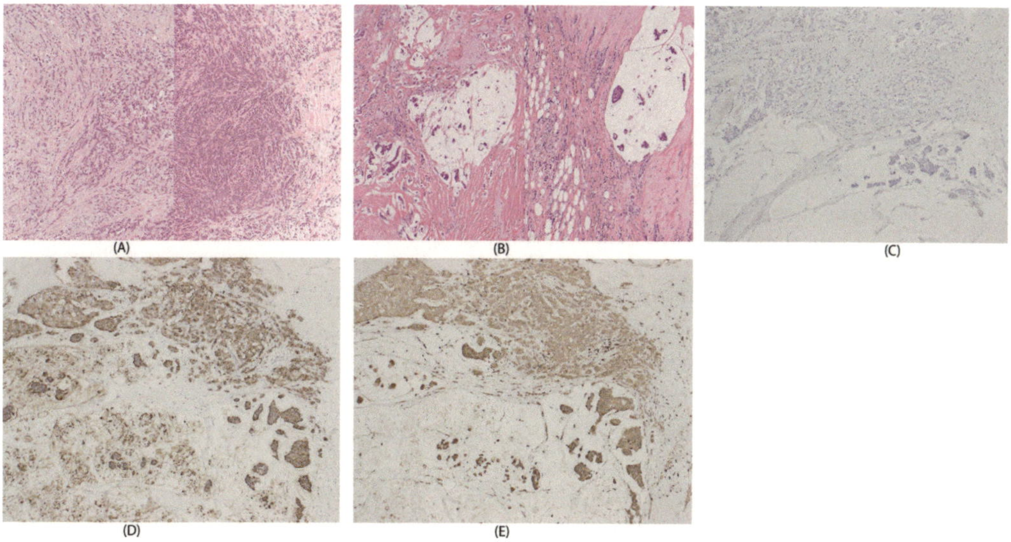

Figure 4. (A) The neoplastic cells are arranged in files or cords infiltrating the stroma. Partially, trabecular type lesion is observed. (B) Within the tumor, there are areas showing atypical cells floating in a pool of mucin. (C) All the tumor cells are negative for E-cadherin immunostaining. (D) All the tumor cells and extracellular mucin are MUC1 positive. (E) All the tumor cells and extracellular mucin are MUC3 positive.

4. Discussion

The major types of invasive carcinomas are categorized as ductal carcinoma. Invasive lobular carcinoma is the second most common histological type of breast carcinoma, accounting for about 5–15% of all invasive breast cancers [14, 15]. Hence, accurate diagnosis of invasive lobular carcinoma is thought to be important. We will discuss about general radiological findings of invasive lobular carcinoma and correlation of our case.

In mammography, Berg et al. [16] examined the performance of mammography as a function of both tumor type and breast density. Mammographic sensitivity was 81% for invasive ductal carcinoma compared with 34% for invasive lobular carcinoma; when only those patients with dense breast tissue were considered, sensitivities decreased dramatically to 60 and 11%, respectively [16]. Because of these diagnostic interests, it is crucial for breast radiologists to be aware of the asymmetric and subtle mammographic features of invasive lobular carcinoma.

A high-density spiculated or irregular margined mass on mammography means invasive carcinoma. Spicula or irregular margin is thought to be invasion of the breast fat tissue and stromal reaction that disrupts normal breast parenchymal architecture. common mammographic manifestations of invasive lobular carcinoma include spiculated or irregular margined mass or asymmetric density. In our case, these findings are not observed. Apart from spiculated, irregular margined masses and asymmetric densities, the most common mammographic manifestation of invasive lobular carcinoma is architectural distortion, which accounts for about 14–25% of cases of mammographically detected invasive lobular carcinoma [3, 17, 18].

Similarly, our case demonstrated architectural distortion on left upper portion in MLO view. We think distortion on mammography means stromal reaction and malignancy.

Ultrasonography of the breast is used primarily as a diagnostic imaging tool. The most common sonographic appearance of invasive lobular carcinoma is a low-echoic mass with posterior acoustic shadowing occurring in up to 60% of cases, however, posterior acoustic shadowing may be lacking in up to 20% of cases [19]. The present case of ultrasonographical findings is thought to be concordant with report of Karen et al. [19].

Here, we will discuss correlation between MRI findings and pathological findings. Our case of mammographic and ultrasonographic findings suggested the possibility of malignancy. Therefore, magnetic resonance imaging (MRI) of 1.5T (Philips) was performed. On MRI, diffusion-weighted image of b-value 1000 s/mm^2 showed mass-like high signal intensity. Apparent diffusion coefficient (ADC)-map revealed diffusion limitation of the water molecule. Besides, irregular shaped and margined mass was observed in T1 weighted image. These findings suggest malignancy in our case. Furthermore, this finding is similar to the report of Mann et al. of invasive lobular carcinoma [6]. Fat-saturated T2 weighted image of the mass showed small high signal intensity area within the mass. This finding suggests the tumor associated mucinous lesion or coexistence of mucinous carcinoma. However, Rosa et al. [9] reported signet-ring cells floating in a pool of mucinous areas (extracellular mucinous lesion) represented at the most 20% of the tumor. We think this extracellular mucin area is not so large but a small area. If invasive carcinoma and mucinous carcinoma are coexisted as collision tumor, the mucinous area which shows very high signal intensity on T2 weighted image would be larger. In our case, extracellular mucin area was approximately 10% of the tumor. This small area of high signal intensity on T2 weighted image might be one of the specific features of invasive lobular carcinoma with extracellular mucin. Dynamic-curve of the contrast-enhanced MRI showed rapid washout pattern. Rapid washout pattern is also seen in invasive ductal or lobular carcinoma. ADC value was 0.577×10^{-3} mm^2/s, hence the existence of water restriction was suggested. From these findings, dynamic-curve, diffusion-weighted image, and ADC-map were suggestive for malignant tumor. And contrast-enhanced T1 weighted image of irregular shaped and margined mass was indicative of invasive carcinoma such as invasive ductal carcinoma or invasive lobular carcinoma. T2 weighted image of small high signal intensity area is thought to be mucinous carcinoma or mucin production. And mucin production is known to be associated with neuroendocrine differentiation. Taking these findings into consideration, other differential diagnoses of this tumor were (i) mixed mucinous-ductal carcinoma, (ii) mucinous carcinoma with neuroendocrine feature, (iii) mucinous papillary neoplasms, and (iv) carcinoma of mixed type (lobular and ductal carcinoma). However, histopathological findings revealed the tumor was composed of single cell with moderate pleomorphism and lack of cohesion. The neoplastic cells were arranged in files or cords infiltrating the stroma. In situ lesion of the invasive lobular carcinoma was not observed. The multifocality of cancer lesion was not demonstrated. Within the tumor, there were areas showing signet-ring cells floating in a pool of mucin. The presence of extracellular mucin is not characteristic of lobular carcinomas. Therefore, immunohistochemical stain for E-cadherin was performed. However, the lesions were completely negative for E-cadherin immunostaining. E-cadherin, a cell-cohesion protein encoded by a gene on chromosome 16q22.1, is the current marker of choice to help discriminate between lobular and ductal carcinoma [11]. Neuroendocrine marker of synaptophysin immunostaining was also negative. Hence, final diagnosis of our tumor is invasive ductal carcinoma with extracellular mucin. From the results of MRI findings, irregular shaped and margined mass with small area of fat-saturated T2 high signal intensity might be one of the special feature of invasive lobular carcinoma with extracellular mucin. Our case is the fourth case in the English literature. Because the number of cases of these tumors is limited, it is difficult to comment on the biological behavior and molecular profiles. However, this diagnosis is important for prognosis and management, and further examination is needed.

In our case, estrogen receptor (ER), progesterone receptor (PgR), and human epidermal growth factor receptor 2 (HER2) status were 99, 0%, and negative, respectively. Invasive lobular carcinoma is known to be more commonly estrogen receptor-positive and HER2-negative, in other words, invasive lobular carcinoma is usually categorized as luminal subtype. The previous reports of Rosa et al. and Haltas et al. [9, 11] are ER positive of luminal subtype. Our case is concordant with their results. However, the results of Yu et al. [10] were not only ER-positive but also HER2 strongly positive. They thought that this type of HER2 status demonstrate various features.

The spectrum of breast lesions that demonstrate extracellular mucin includes fibrocystic change with luminal mucin, mucocele-like lesions, papillary lesions with mucin secretion, and mucinous carcinoma among others [9]. In contrast, lobular neoplasia and invasive lobular carcinoma demonstrate intracytoplasmic mucin, and no cases of lobular carcinoma with extracellular mucin have been found except previous three reports [9–11, 20].

Invasive lobular carcinoma comprises 5–15% of invasive breast tumors [14, 15]. They can occur at any age. The median age at diagnosis is between 45 and 56 years and there is a tendency to affect older patients compared with ductal carcinoma [8, 9], similar to our results of the 77-year-old. The presenting symptom in most cases is a mass with irregular margins or a breast thickening with diffuse nodularity [8, 9]. The clinical features of invasive lobular carcinoma are also different from that of ductal carcinomas. Invasive lobular carcinomas tend to be more often multifocal and bilateral [8, 9], with a distinct metastatic pattern and a higher frequency of bone, gastrointestinal tract, uterus, meninges, and diffuse serosal involvement [21]. Hence, discrimination between lobular carcinoma and ductal carcinoma is important clinically, radiologically, and pathologically. In our case, multifocality of the tumor was not observed similarly to the reports of Rosa et al. and Yu et al. [9, 10]. However, the case of Haltas et al. [11] indicated multifocality. We think this is because the variant of invasive lobular carcinoma with extracellular mucin might present different behavior compared with classical invasive lobular carcinoma.

Mucin has been classified as membrane-bound mucin, which mediates signal transduction, and secretary mucin, which are directly secreted into extracellular spaces. In the MUC immunostaining family, the membrane-bound mucins include MUC1, MUC3, MUC4, and the secretary mucins include MUC2, MUC5AC, MUC6 [22]. In our current case, MUC4, MUC5AC, and MUC6 were negative; however, all the tumor cells revealed cytoplasmic expression of MUC1. Molecular and biochemical studies have demonstrated that MUC1 is involved in the inhibition of E-cadherin mediated -cell and cell-matrix adhesion [10, 22–25]. The cytoplasmic domain of MUC1 molecule has been shown to inhibit the formation of E-cadherin-β-catenin complex [10, 24]. Therefore MUC1 may play a role in tumor invasion and metastases by disrupting cell adhesions [10]. Similarly, our case of tumor invasion may correlate with the MUC1 cytoplasmic expression.

Additionally, our case of all the tumor cells was positive for MUC3 immunostaining. Rakha et al. and Furuya et al. [26, 27] reported that MUC3 immunostaining is useful for distinguishing between benign lesion and malignant lesion of the breast carcinoma. Our case is concordant with their reports, and membrane-bound mucin of MUC3 may mediate signal transduction correlate with malignancy. Furthermore, Rakha et al. [26] indicated that most breast carcinomas express MUC1, MUC3, and MUC4; however, MUC1 and MUC3 are potential prognostic indicators. Hence, diagnosing invasive lobular carcinoma with extracellular mucin is important on not only pathologically but also radiologically.

Early genomic studies revealed very little overall difference in genomic profiles between low-grade invasive ductal carcinoma and classical invasive lobular carcinoma, implying that classical invasive lobular carcinoma might represent a subtype of low-grade invasive ductal carcinoma [10]. Recent gene expression studies comparing invasive lobular carcinoma and invasive ductal carcinoma have identified two subsets of invasive lobular carcinoma with distinct transcription patterns [10]. Approximately, half of the invasive lobular carcinomas differs from invasive ductal carcinomas in gene expression profiles ("typical" invasive lobular carcinomas), while the remaining invasive lobular carcinomas closely resemble invasive ductal carcinomas in transcription patterns. ("ductal-like" invasive lobular carcinomas) [10]. On the other hand, a recent study on grade- and molecular subtype-matched invasive lobular carcinomas and invasive ductal carcinomas of no special type demonstrated that invasive lobular carcinomas had different transcriptomic profiles in the genes related to cell-to-cell adhesion and signaling, as well as actin cytoskeleton signaling, when compared with grade- and molecular subtype-matched invasive ductal carcinomas [10]. This finding suggested that even though invasive lobular carcinomas and invasive ductal carcinomas might present as a spectrum or form of a family [10]. Taking into consideration of the above Yu et al. reported case, our current case might be in the middle stage of the spectrum between lobular carcinoma and ductal carcinoma. We think existence of extracellular mucin is not definitive for ductal phenotype not only histologically but also genetically.

5. Conclusion

We encountered the distinct variant of invasive lobular carcinoma with extracellular mucin. We described the correlation of its radiological and pathological interest. Radiological findings of invasive lobular carcinoma with extracellular mucin are documented in English literature for the first time. We suggest one of the MRI special features of our case is not only irregular shaped and margined mass but also small T2-high-signal intensity. These findings by the knowledge from radiopathological correlation might be one of the specific features of invasive lobular carcinoma with extracellular mucin. Further examinations are needed to clarify this lesion.

Acknowledgements

We thank Shigeko Ohnuma and Manabu Kubota department of the St. Marianna University of pathology for their technical assistance and advices.

Author details

Shinya Tajima[1,2]*, Keiko Kishimoto[2], Yoshihide Kanemaki[2], Ichiro Maeda[1], Akira Endo[1], Motohiro Chosokabe[1], Takafumi Ono[2], Koichiro Tsugawa[3] and Masayuki Takagi[1]

*Address all correspondence to: stajima0829@gmail.com

1 Department of Pathology and Radiology, St. Marianna University School of Medicine, Kawasaki City, Kanagawa, Japan

2 Department of Radiology, St. Marianna University School of Medicine, Kawasaki City, Kanagawa, Japan

3 Department of Breast and Endocrine Surgery, St. Marianna University School of Medicine, Kawasaki City, Kanagawa, Japan

References

[1] Mendelson EB, Harris KM, Doshi N, et al. Infiltrating lobulacarcinoma: Mammographic patteforrns with pathologic correlation. American Journal of Radiology. 1989;**153**:265-271

[2] Helvie MA, Paramagul C, Oberman HA, et al. Invasive lobular carcinoma imaging features and clinical detection. Investigative Radiology. 1993;**28**:202-207

[3] Le GM, Ollivier L, Asselain B, et al. Mammographic features of 455 invasive lobular carcinomas. Radiology. 1992;**185**:705-708

[4] White JR, Gustafson GS, Wimbish K, et al. Conservative surgery and radiation therapy for infiltrating lobular carcinoma of the breast. The role of preoperative mammograms in guiding treatment. Cancer. 1994;**74**:640-647

[5] Butler RS, Venta LA, Wiley EL, et al. Sonographic evaluation of infiltrating lobular carcinoma. American Journal of Roentgenology. 1999;**172**:325-330

[6] Mann RM, Hoogeveen YL, Blickman JG, et al. MRI compared to conventional diagnostic work-up in the detection and evaluation of invasive lobular carcinoma of the breast: A review of existing literature. Breast Cancer Research and Treatment. 2008;**107**:1-14

[7] Foote FW Jr, Stewart FW. A histologic classification of carcinoma of the breast. Surgery. 1946;**19**:74-99

[8] Rosen PP. Invasive lobular carcinoma. In: Rosen's Breast Pathology. 3rd ed. Philadelphia, PA: Lippincott Williams and Wilkins; 2001. pp. 690-705

[9] Rosa M, Mohammadi A, Masood S. Lobular carcinoma of the breast with extracellular mucin: New variant of mucin-producing carcinoma? Pathology International. 2009;**59**:405-409

[10] Yu J, Bhargava R, Dabbs DJ. Invasive lobular carcinoma with extracellular mucin production and HER-2 overexpression: A case report and further case studies. Diagnostic Pathology. 2010;**5**:36

[11] Haltas H, Bayrak R, Yenidunya S, et al. Invasive lobular carcinoma with extracellular mucin as a distinct variant of lobular carcinoma: A case report. Diagnostic Pathology. 2012;**7**:91

[12] D'Orsi CJ, Sickles EA, Mendelson EB, et al, editors. ACR BI-RADS Atlas Breast Imaging Reporting and Data System. 5th ed. Reston, VA: American College of Radiology; 2013

[13] Tozaki M, Fukuma E. MR spectroscopy and diffusion weighted imaging of the breast: Are they useful tools for characterizing breast lesions before biopsy?. American Journal of Roentgenology. 2009;**193**:840-809

[14] Sastre-Garau X, Jouve M, Asselain B, et al. Infiltrating lobular carcinoma of the breast. Clinicopathologic analysis of 975 cases with reference to data on conservative therapy and metastatic patterns. Cancer. 1996;**77**:113-120

[15] Borst MJ, Ingold JA. Metastatic patterns of invasive lobular versus invasive ductal carcinoma of the breast. Surgery. 1993;**144**:637-641

[16] Berg WA, Gutierrez L, NessAiver MS, et al. Diagnostic accuracy of mammography, clinical examination, US, and MR imaging in preoperative assessment of breast cancer. Radiology. 2004;**233**:830-849

[17] Hilleren DJ, Andersson IT, Lindholm K, et al. Invasive lobular carcinoma: Mammographic findings in a 10-year experience. Radiology. 1991;**178**:149-154

[18] Krecke KN, Gisvold JJ. Invasive lobular carcinoma of the breast: Mammographic findings and extent of disease at diagnosis in 184 patients. American Journal of Roentgenology. 1993;**161**:957-960

[19] Karen J, Deba S, Shelley EH. Lobular breast cancer series: imaging. Breast Cancer Research. 2015;**17**:94

[20] Tan PH, Tse GM, Bay BH. Mucinous breast lesions: Diagnostic challenges. Journal of Clinical Pathology. 2008;**61**:11-19

[21] Ellis OI, Schnitt SJ, Sastre-Garau X, et al. Invasive breast carcinoma. In: Tavassoli FA, Devillee P, editors. Tumours of the Breast and Female Genital Organs. Lyon: IARC Press; 2003. pp. 23-25, 48-49

[22] Singh PK, Hollingsworth MA. Cell surface-associated mucins in signal transduction. Trends in Cell Biology. 2006;**16**:467-476

[23] Rahn JJ, Dabbagh L, Pasdar M, et al. The importance of MUC1 cellular localization in patients with breast carcinoma: An immunohistologic study of 71 patients and review of the literature. Cancer. 2001;**91**:1973-1982

[24] Kondo K, Kohno N, Yokoyama A, et al. Decreased MUC1 expression induces E-cadherin-mediated cell adhesion of breast cancer cell lines. Cancer Research. 1998;**58**:2014-2019

[25] Wesseling J, van der Valk SW, Hilkens J. A mechanism for inhibition of E-cadherin-mediated cell-cell adhesion by the membrane-associated mucin episialin/MUC1. Molecular Biology of the Cell. 1996;**7**:565-577

[26] Rakha EA, Boyce RWG, El-Rehim DA, et al. Expression of mucins (MUC1, MUC2, MUC3, MUC4, MUC5AC and MUC6) and their prognostic significance in human breast cancer. Modern Pathology. 2005;**18**:1295-1304

[27] Furuya C, Kawano H, Yamanouchi T, et al. Combined evaluation of CK5/6, ER, p63, and MUC3 for distinguishing breast intraductal papilloma from ductal carcinoma in situ. Pathology International. 2012;**62**:381-390

Chapter 2

Near-Field Radar Microwave Imaging as an Add-on Modality to Mammography

Ashkan Ghanbarzadeh Dagheyan, Ali Molaei,
Richard Obermeier, Aida K. Martinez and
Jose Martinez Lorenzo

Additional information is available at the end of the chapter

http://dx.doi.org/10.5772/intechopen.69726

Abstract

According to global statistics, there is a high incidence of cancer in western countries; and, due to the limited resources available in most health care systems, it seems like one of the most feasible options to fight against cancer might be strict prevention policies—such as eliminating carcinogens in people's daily lives. Nevertheless, early cancer detection and effective treatment are still necessary, and understanding their efficacy and limitations are important issues that need to be addressed in order to ultimately enhance patients' survival rate. In the case of breast cancer, some of the problems faced by conventional mammography have been addressed in the literature; they include high rate of false-positive and false-negative results, as well as the possibility of overdiagnosis. New technologies, such as digital breast tomosynthesis (DBT), have been able to improve the sensitivity and specificity by using 3D imaging. However, the low contrast (1%) existing between tumors and healthy fibroglandular tissue at X-ray frequencies has been identified as one of the main causes of misdiagnosis in both conventional 2D mammography and DBT. Near-field radar imaging (NRI) provides a unique opportunity to overcome this problem, since the contrast existing between the aforementioned tissues is intrinsically higher (10%) at microwave frequencies. Moreover, the low resolution and highly complex scattering patterns of microwave systems can be enhanced by using prior information from other modalities, such as the DBT. Therefore, a multimodal DBT/NRI imaging system is proposed to exploit their individual strengths while minimizing their weaknesses. In this work, the foundation of this idea is reviewed, and a preliminary design and experimental validation of the NRI system, used as a DBT complement, is introduced.

Keywords: breast cancer detection, microwave imaging, near-field radar imaging, antipodal Vivaldi antennas, digital breast tomosynthesis, breast cancer statistics

1. Introduction

According to the most recent statistics from SEER [1], around 14, 140, 254 individuals were living with a type of cancer in 2013; and, based on the 2011–2013 data, approximately 39% of men and women will be diagnosed with cancer during their lifetime in the US [1]. Particularly, breast cancer is the most prevalent cancer in terms of incidence, and it is the second cause of cancer death among women after bronchus cancer [2]. Furthermore, the data from 1975 to 2013 illustrates that the incidence of breast cancer has had either an ascending or irregular trend across almost all races in the US. Mostly due to advancements in detection and treatment, the rate of mortality has decreased. However, looking at the incidence statistics, it is clear that the efforts in preventing breast cancer can still be improved [1, 3]. Environmental factors such as exposure to ionizing radiation, inheriting certain genes such as BRCA1 and BRCA2, and, most importantly, lifestyle have been associated with an increase in the risk of breast cancer. For instance, the link between breast carcinogenesis and naturally occurring substances such as heterocyclic amines (HCAs), insulin-like growth hormone (IGF-I), animal estrogen (E2), and bovine leukaemia virus (BLV), which are ubiquitous in western and modern diets, have been substantiated with a vast body of evidence [4–11]. Nonetheless, not much has been done in updating the dietary guidelines and food policies to address the role of these substances, and similar ones, in cancer epidemic. In parallel, statistics show that, in general, the rate of breast cancer and other types of cancer are appreciably higher in western and industrialized countries [12], which can be attributed to both advanced detection technologies and lifestyle. The experience from Japan's transition towards adopting a western diet and the dramatic increase in cancer and Alzheimer's disease rates [13–15] as well as Japanese-American immigrants' higher risk of cancer compared to the people residing in Japan [16], are in accordance with the mentioned statistics. Similar observations have been made in the case of ischemic heart diseases [16, 17] and Alzheimer's disease [18] in other countries. These studies report that (1) in some countries such as Uganda coronary heart diseases only happened in rare cases, in contrast to the global trend in which ischemic heart disease is the number one cause of death; and (2) despite the high frequency of Alzheimer's genes (APO E 4 allele) in countries such as Nigeria, the disease itself is not as nearly prevalent as in western countries. **Figure 1** recapitulates the aforementioned statistics of breast cancer. Until interventions are made to eliminate the possible causes of breast cancer–and cancer in overall–and to seriously implement prevention programs, early detection via imaging and other screening tools and advanced treatment techniques are probably the only temporary solutions to address this matter.

One of the new early detection methods for breast cancer that has attracted much attention during the last decade is near-field radar imaging (NRI) with microwaves. Though microwave imaging is limited by low resolution, it can provide additional information about the breast composition, since the contrast between malignant and healthy fibroglandular tissues at microwave frequencies is more than that at X-ray frequencies. This chapter is aimed at describing a microwave imaging system that can be added to digital breast tomosynthesis (DBT), also a novel 3D X-ray machine, to make possible a bimodal screening method. Firstly, the shortcomings of mammography as the most widely used screening method is briefly reviewed to show the necessity of introducing novel and more accurate breast imaging methods. Then, the

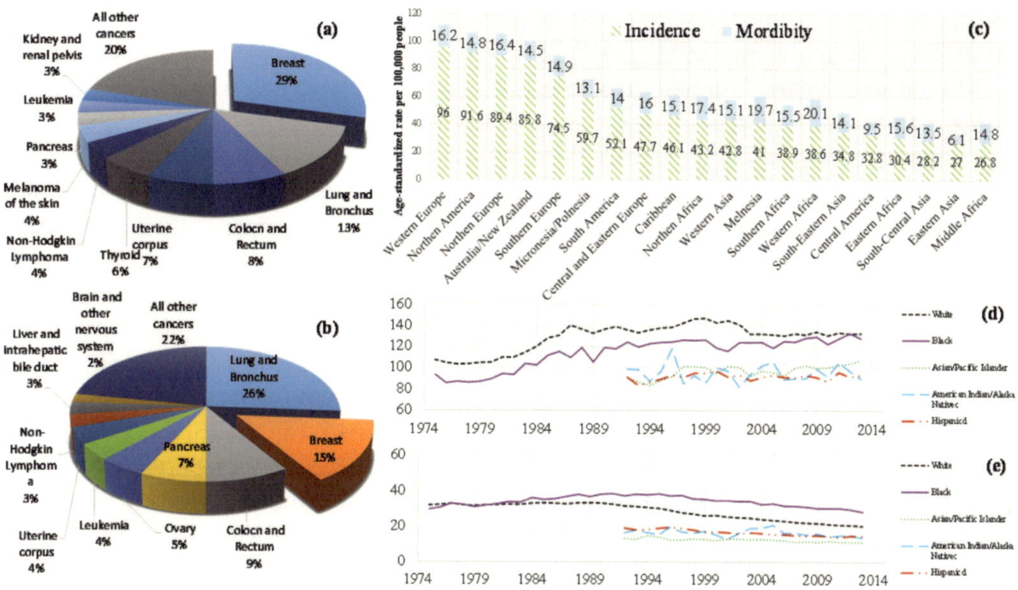

Figure 1. Breast cancer statistics in the US and the globe at glance: (a) Incidence and (b) mortality rate with respect to other types of cancer in the US, (c) incidence and mortality rate compared among a number of countries, (d) incidence and (e) mortality rates in the US from 1975 to 2013.

possible benefits and details of adding a near-field imaging system to X-ray mammography is discussed. It is predicted that the final bimodal, NIR-X-ray (DBT), imaging system has the potential to improve true-positive (TP) diagnosis.

2. Drawbacks of mammography

Mammography, as the most widely used modality for population-based breast cancer screening, employs X-ray radiation to reconstruct images of the breast. Inspite of the 34% reduction in breast cancer morbidity rate [19] attributed mainly to advancements in detection and treatment, more research is yet needed to find more effective imaging and treatment methods. Despite the contributions of mammography to this reduction, the possibility of false-positive results, false-negative results, and overdiagnosis associated with it, as addressed in the literature, has raised some substantiated concerns. These three inherent shortcomings of current X-ray imaging technology are briefly reviewed in the following subsections.

2.1. False-positive results

A false-positive (FP) outcome is referred to a case where the breast is actually cancer-free, but the mammogram is misread as abnormal. In the New England study in 2000, the risk of obtaining an FP result was estimated to be 6.5%, and it was reported that at least 23.8% of the study participants received an FP result [20]. The risk could go up as high as 43.1% after nine mammograms. Another study reported a prevalence of 10.6% of FP results among women in the age range of 50–51 in their first mammography session. In the following sessions, the probability was approximated to be 3.8%; but the cumulative risk of getting an FP outcome turned out to be 32.4%, implying that one out of three women could receive an FP alarm during a 10-year biannual screening program [21]. The large study performed in 2011 reported that there is a prevalence of 16.3 and 9.6% in obtaining an FP result in the first and following sessions, severally. The cumulative risk was found to be 61.3% for women starting their regular session at the age of 40 or 50, in an annual screening program [22]. Before the possibility of breast cancer is ruled out, a patient who receives a positive result is recalled for further examination that usually includes ultrasound imaging, needle biopsy, and sometimes surgical biopsies. These biopsies, which some authors call "unnecessary" [23, 24], as well as the prolonged uncertainty about ones' health status, can be accompanied by a psychological trauma similar to those who were diagnosed with cancer in their first 6 months with symptoms such as short-term anxiety, more frequent self-examinations, and a change in the patients' tendency to attend later mammography sessions [25–28]. It has also been reported that 27 and 33% of women gone under breast biopsy had reduced sexual sensitivity and pain in the breast. In addition, an increment in mood disturbances and reduction in natural killer cell activity and INF γ production was observed before and after biopsy [26, 27]. Therefore, FP results can lead to serious consequences that need to be addressed.

2.2. False-negative results

As the name implies, when a malignant tissue is not detected in a mammogram, the result is a false-negative (FN). The tumor might be detected in the next screening sessions, when perhaps it has grown visible due to invasion into the encompassing tissues. The data on the prevalence of FN results has been inconsistent. In a 1996 study, it was found that, depending on family history, follow-up duration, and age; between 12.5 and 31.5% of mammograms were interpreted as cancer-free, while there was actually a tumor in the breast [29]. A more recent study, in 2014, showed that FN probability in digital and screen-film mammography for women above (under) 50 was 24% (27%) and 27% (24%), respectively [30]. It was reported that obtaining an FN result was directly associated with breast density. Other factors that play a role in FN evaluation of breast are the type of cancer (particularly BRCA 1 and BRCA 2 mutations) and the location of the tumor (being close to the chest wall) [31, 32].

2.3. Overdiagnosis

Overdiagnosis may be defined as "the detection of cases that would never have come to clinical attention without screening [in a patient's lifetime] [32]." Though some physicians disagree with the numbers reported for such cases [33]. Some studies from 2004 reported overdiagnosis rates of 5% in ductile carcinoma *in situ* (DCIS) in Italy [33] and 33% in general mammography of women of ages 50–59 in Norway and Sweden [34]. The results from the later study were comparable with the 30% rate of overdiagnosis reported in [35], back in 2001. A larger study in 2005, which was carried out over eleven counties in Sweden, reported the risk of overdiagnosis as 21 and 54% for women in age groups of 50–59 and 60–69, in order [37]. The prevalence of subclinical tumors among women after 50 was explained as the reason for rather high risks of overdiagnosis. On the other hand, a recent report in 2015 from South

Australia reported the overdiagnosis risk as 8% for invasive cancer and 12% for when cases of DCIS were included in the data [36]. Also, a review on studies conducted in European countries reported the risk to be 1–10% [37]. The discrepancies in numbers reported by different researchers is illustrative of the complexities involved in estimating breast cancer overdiagnosis.

Based on the problems described in this section, the necessity of investigating new science and developing novel technologies for breast imaging, either as complementary or standalone modalities, is evident. The focus of the work presented in this chapter is on reducing false-positive and false-negative results by fusing the information acquired by two different modalities. However, overdiagnosis cannot be addressed with the current status of the add-on NRI unit.

3. Digital breast tomosynthesis (DBT)

About 40% of eligible women who are recommended to have regular screening have dense breasts, which are composed of more than 50% glandular tissue and are among the major contributors to uncertain mammogram readings [38, 39]. Thereby, one of the focuses of new screening devices is to enable better imaging visibility through different layers of breast. This is not properly addressed in conventional 2D mammograms of the breast; since an existing tumor can be masked by underlying and overlying tissues and, thus, make accurate diagnosis difficult for radiologists. In order to enhance the image resolution, full-field digital mammography (FFDM) detectors can be utilized. The DBT employs these detectors as well as a rotating X-ray tube that moves in a circular arc to illuminate the breast from different angles [40]. Then, images of several 2D projections at dissimilar depths are reconstructed, making it feasible for radiologists to look through different layers. Aside from hardware enhancements, novel imaging algorithms –including, but not limited to, filtered back projection and Gaussian frequency blending; and iterative techniques such as Maximum Likelihood and Simultaneous Algebraic Reconstruction Technique—have been applied in the DBT on the software level [40].

Conventional mammography makes use of film-screening, which provides high resolution to delineate micro-calcifications and other fine features in the breast; yet, it has a narrow dynamic range that limits tumor visualization in dense segments of the breast. FFDM, however, improves dynamic range and provides the radiologists with the option to manipulate the reconstructed images. Moreover, higher contrast is observed between dense glandular and fatty tissue when FFDM detectors are used [40]. The efficacy of the DBT has been put to the test to evaluate how effective its new features are in practice. In a study in 2005, it was reported that for the age group under 50, premenopausal women, and patients with consistently or extremely dense breasts; the accuracy of images acquired by digital mammography was higher than that of conventional mammography [41]. Additionally, it was shown that the margin, calcification, and lesion visibility of the DBT was superior to conventional imaging in the images of an FDA-certified breast phantom. The radiation exposure levels were similar or less in the DBT; and the tumor boundaries and vessels around calcifications were clearer, which contribute to better identification of malignant and benign masses [42]. Based on the better lesion visibility of the DBT, Teersa et al. recommended tomosynthesis as a complementary modality to 2D mammography [42]. The combination of 3D and 2D mammography is more commonly adopted than 3D imaging alone in clinical settings [40].

The improved accuracy using 2D-3D mammography was also observed by Bernardi et al. [43, 44]. Better visualization of tumors, as provided by a 2D-3D setup could reduce the number of FP results and consequently result in fewer follow-up biopsies. Consistent with this prediction, in 2009, Gur and others reported 10% decrease in false-positives when DBT was used in addition to FFDM [45]. In a more recent study in 2014, the ascendency of 2D-3D mammography over 2D mammography was substantiated in terms of true-positive evaluation and sensitivity [46]. In the same year, Bernardi's subsequent study showed a considerable elevation, from 60% in 2D to 87% in true-positive readings of radiologists when using a 2D-3D configuration [47]. One year later, Svahns et al. considered the FP to TP ratios in three population-based studies and reported improvements in radiologists' interpretive efficacy of X-ray images when a combined configuration was implemented. The results indicated 55, 48 and 30% improvement in true positive detection when a 2D-3D setup was used in lieu of traditional setup in Houston, STORM, and Oslo studies, severally [48]. In TOMMY trial in UK, 2015, increased specificity (by 9%) for all studied groups and elevated sensitivity (by 7%) for dense breasts was observed as a result of using digital and film screening [49]. A 2016 review also reported fewer recall rates using the DBT [50].

4. Breast near-field radar imaging (NRI)

4.1. Background

The contrast between cancerous and fibroglandular tissues is higher when they are exposed to microwave radiation than when they are illuminated by X-ray [53]. This contrast is increased about 5–10 fold when moving form X-ray to microwave frequencies, contingent upon the operating frequency span [51, 52], which renders microwave imaging a distinct candidate to be used as a complementary modality to 2D-3D mammography. A large study by Lazebnik et al. showed that the difference between dielectric properties of malignant and normal tissue is 10% when the fibroglandular tissue is in the background and 10:1 when the adipose-dominant tissue is considered as reference [53]. Though the former is significantly lower than the adipose/tumor contrast, it is still remarkably higher than the fibroglandular/tumor contrast in X-ray frequencies, which is about 1% [54]. **Figure 2** displays the *ex vivo* tissue properties as reported in [53] and as can be observed, the dissimilarity between the fibroglandular and malignant tissue is appreciable. Halter et al. showed that the difference between the dielectric properties of healthy and malignant tissues measured *in vivo*, using microwave and electrical impedance spectroscopy during reduction surgeries, is decreased [54]. However, the contrast is still adequately large for NRI to be a technique of interest as an improvement to conventional or digital mammography. Meaney et al. also pointed out that even though the *in vivo* measurements exhibit lower microwave contrast of about 2:1 (tumor permittivity: average permittivity of breast) at 0.9 GHz, the difference is still significant compared to that in most other traditional imaging systems [52]. Besides high complex permittivity values, there are other features that

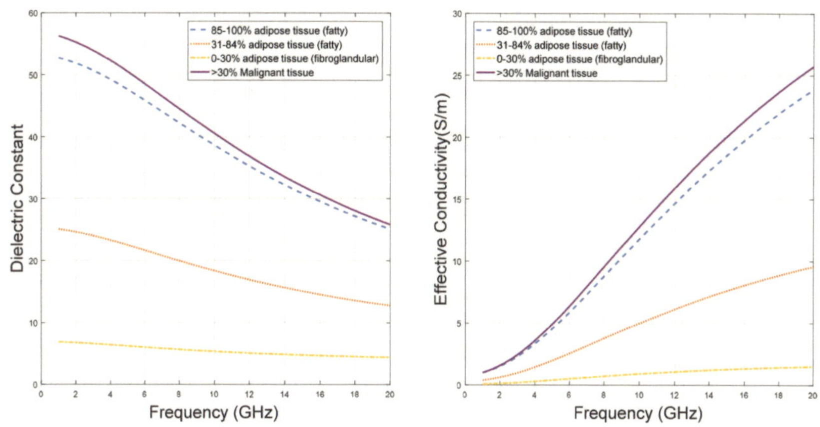

Figure 2. Comparison between the dielectric properties and conductivity of healthy tissues and malignant tissues. Plots are based on the data from [53].

make NRI a suitable candidate for breast screening. It is intrinsically non-ionizing and it does not require breast compression when used independently. Also, microwave imaging provides high sensitivity for revealing small-sized masses. These qualities come at a considerably lower cost than other methods such as nuclear medicine and magnetic resonance imaging (MRI) [55].

To be able to reconstruct images of breast in microwave frequencies, several studies have been dedicated to find practical imaging algorithms including [56–58] that introduce finite difference time-domain (FDTD) and finite element techniques. Among other introduced methods, iterative numerical techniques such as conjugate gradient least square, Newton-Kantorovish, and Levenberg-Marquardt [59–61]; as well as finite difference frequency-domain (FDFD) can be mentioned [62–67]. The moderate imaging resolution in current clinical layouts can be enhanced via novel algorithms such as solving the 3D inverse problem employing variable-strength spatial prior constraints [66] and applying compressive sensing confocal imaging algorithms [67]. Both of these methods present encouraging results for the future of NRI. Making use of prior geometry or information, acquired by other imaging modalities, for microwave imaging is an ongoing research subject that can facilitate breast tomography and image reconstruction. Two recent works in this area used microwave radar imaging and MRI to feed the dielectric parameter reconstruction codes with spatial information. Baran et al. restored the average dielectric properties of different tissue types by microwave radar imaging and then used the data to perform microwave tomography [68]. They were able to obtain finer reconstruction qualities using this hybrid method than when tomography and radar-based imaging were conducted separately. Golnabi et al. employed an MRI image to reconstruct the complex permittivity of a real breast [69]. They reported improved accuracy and contrast between the target and background medium that were fibroglandular and adipose tissues, respectively. One year later, in 2016, they implemented this idea in a 3D reconstruction and again achieved promising outcomes with up to 2 and 9 times improvement in accuracy of conductivity and permittivity maps, respectively [70]. Due to the interference of metallic parts with the magnetic fields, combining microwave imaging and MRI in the same physical setup was reported to be unfeasible.

4.2. Breast NRI at experimental level

One of the first NRI system implementable for a clinical trial was introduced in 2000 by Meaney and his colleagues [52]. The operational bandwidth of the system was 0.3–1 GHz and it was configured in a way that a patient could comfortably lie down on a bed with her breast pendent in a liquid inside a container with a circular antenna array encompassing the breast. The antennas were immersed in the same liquid (saline) as the matching medium, and they collected the scattered field from the submerged breast from multiple directions. The scan took 10–15 min for each breast of the human participants of the trial, using a tomographic method from the chest to the nipple. As predicted, the reconstructed maps of dielectric properties were of low resolution; however, they showed that the *in vivo* breast properties are larger than the ones obtained from *ex vivo* measurements. Later in 2007, the same group reported a good agreement between images retrieved by microwave imaging and MRI from subjects with normal mammograms and multiple phantoms [66]. Particularly, it was shown that fibroglandular tissue distribution and water content agreed well between the two sets of images. Furthermore, they found that similar to fat percentage and density, dielectric properties of the breast are heterogeneous.

Klemm et al. assembled a similar physical setup except, in place of a circular antenna, they used a set of ultra-wideband (UWB) antennas that were arranged in a hemispherical shape to conform to the shape of the pendent breast [71]. The system's performance was evaluated based on experiments carried out on a phantom encapsulated in a shell mimicking skin. They were able to detect small tumor simulants, 4-6 mm in diameter, embedded in the phantoms by implementing two beamforming algorithms, multi-static microwave imaging (MAMI) and delay-and-sum (DAS). Later, the system was tested on highly heterogeneous phantoms and it was shown to give promising results [72]. Also, in a clinical case study, the system was tested on a real breast, and the obtained image was compared to its associated mammogram. The malignant tissue was correctly located in the microwave image when compared to the X-ray image [73].

Lai and his group also employed UWB antennas to scan a number of heterogeneous and homogenous breast phantoms at Nanyan Technological University [74]. By rotating the phantoms 360 degrees, the antennas simulated a circular set of 360 elements. This configuration enabled them to detect a 4 mm tumor in all phantom types. But, detectability was not strong enough to delineate 2 mm inclusions. Lazero et al. published the results of what they named a "worst-case-study" utilizing a single UWB monopole antenna [75]. The phantom model was filled with water (presenting high losses), with a rod submerged inside it, and the antenna was located in air (presenting high reflection). Notwithstanding these challenging conditions, the embedded rod was successfully detected, implementing FDFD and Wiener-filter algorithm that took into account the effect of a simulated skin interface. Chun Yu and colleagues, in a different experimental layout, used an active microwave imaging method to retrieve images of a clay ball, a metallic ball, and a combined arrangement of both when they were submerged in water [76]. They utilized a dipole single transmitter and receiver to avert the mutual coupling that exists in an antenna array. The transmitting and receiving array were moved by an automatic positioner to enable a flexible, multi-view data acquisition in three dimensions over the surface of the object being measured. Applying an active, hybrid-inversion, reconstruction method, they were able to image one clay ball and the combined arrangement of two clay balls and one metallic ball.

Henriksson et al. made use of a microwave camera, at 2.45 GHz, to quantitatively restore the dielectric properties of materials [77]. In a quantitative approach, in place of approximations, the non-linear diffraction problem is solved at the cost of heavy computations. In 1990, the planar camera was built for non-invasive hyperthermia control; and later, in 1998, it was put to the test by Franchois on a rotating object inside a liquid container. Henriksson and his colleagues used a similar experimental setup that included two horn antennas. They made a breast-equivalent liquid using a Triton X-100 mixture and placed it inside a rotating tube—the object of interest—to have a more realistic model. Albeit some artifacts were present, the system performed well in reconstructing dielectric maps, using the Newton-Kantorovich algorithm. This camera enables NRI to be carried out in a mammographic configuration [77, 78], one of the key benefits of the approach presented in this chapter. More recently, in 2013, imaging a moving target was also tested in an integrated microwave imaging radar, as in an inverse synthetic array radar, at the University of Padova in Italy [79]. In the assembled setup, a planar antenna, consisting of two monopoles and two feed lines, was fixed on a support frame and it radiated down over the moving phantom. Two stepper motors shifted the target in the horizontal plane in two perpendicular directions. The results demonstrated that the system is capable of detecting two embedded inclusions inside the phantom.

Microwave imaging via space-time (MIST) beamforming has been experimentally implemented on phantoms, seeking to solve both 2D and 3D problem. On the simulation level, Bond et al. used a UWB antenna array to transmit the waves and then employed a beam former to reconstruct images of the backscattered signal energy [80]. In order to downsize the overshadowing impact of the skin-like layer of the MRI breast model they used, they utilized a data-adaptive algorithm to eliminate the dominant backscatter at the skin-breast interface. This approach is efficient in that it generates images only in areas of high background energy, i.e. malignant tissues. In the subsequent year, from the same group, Xi Lu et al. tested the practicality of MIST on 3D physical phantoms [81]. The results in 2D and 3D improved considerably compared to those obtained by simple focusing methods. In the 3D case, the contrast between malignant and normal tissue was observed to be 1.5:1 for a 4-mm tumor, which displayed the strong potential of MIST in disclosing small tumors.

At the end of this subsection, some of the recent works that are different in application or scope from the ones previously introduced can be reviewed to show how the practical aspect of microwave imaging has expanded in last few years. In 2014, Eleutério et al. presented a preliminary study to evaluate NRI in the axilla where sentinel nodes are typically found [82]. The significance of this study was to explore the role of microwave imaging in the estimation of metastasis initiation. Grzegorczyk et al. applied microwave imaging to monitor neoadjuvant chemotherapy, as an economic alternative to MRI and PET [83]. Using a different and compact method, researchers at the University of Manitoba examined the capacity of spintronic microwave sensors in biomedical imaging [84]. They demonstrated that these sensors, though only a fraction of microwave antennas in size, have the ability to detect spherical objects inside a homogenous medium with good resolution. Contrast-enhanced NRI has also become a topic of interest in the recent years. In one of the latest works published in 2016, Bucci et al. used magnetic nanoparticles as contrast agent, and showed their applicability by comparing the simulation and laboratory results [85].

5. A near-field radar imaging system for bimodal applications

In the last two sections, some aspects of mammography, digital tomosynthesis, and microwave imaging were reviewed. The idea of a bimodal system that takes advantage of the strengths of both systems and can potentially compensate some of the drawbacks of each modality makes sense in the case of NRI and DBT. Among the number of other different combinations that has been tested in the last few years, NRI and MRI, optical imaging and DBT, and NRI and ultrasound can be listed. In the first case, the interference of the magnetic fields with the metallic part of the microwave imaging system impeded the simultaneous implementation of the NRI and MRI sensors [86], but in the other two cases, important results such as access to the map of vessels around tumors via the optical modality [87] and detection of very small inclusion [88], down to 1.2 mm, were reported. One of the pragmatic ways by which NRI can be added as a complementary system to the DBT is to design and build a compact NRI system that conforms to the geometry of the DBT and can scan the breast in a co-registered fashion using mechanical motion. This idea is illustrated schematically in **Figure 3**: (1) to conform to the DBT's shape, the NRI system was designed to fit into the compression paddle, (2) to be as compact as possible, a set of antipodal Vivaldi antennas (AVAs) were used as the transducer array, (3) to enable mechanical motion, a two-dimensional motion stage was implemented. In the succeeding subsections, the various parts of the system are described in more details.

5.1. Antipodal Vivaldi antennas (AVAs)

Vivaldi antennas are planar, compact in size, and easy to manufacture [91]. These qualities make Vivaldi antenna a good candidate for use in an add-on NRI system, particularly due to

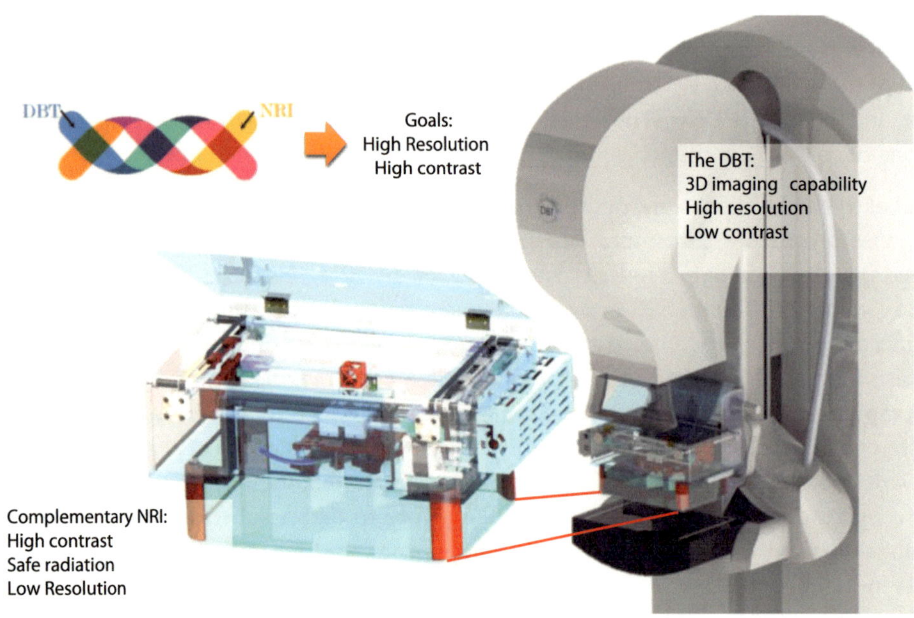

Figure 3. The designed NRI mechatronic system (left) that fits into the compression paddle of the DBT (right). In this manner, first the DBT and then the NRI system scans the breast.

that a number of these antennas can fit into a small space [89]. On the other hand, Vivaldi antennas are limited in bandwidth since they require a balun to convert the micro-strip into a strip-line. One solution to remove this obstacle is to employ antipodal vivaldi antenna (AVAs) that have direct feeding micro-strip lines while maintaining the advantages of Vivaldi antennas. To further reduce the size of the AVAs and improve the coupling of electromagnetic waves going into the breast tissue, they can be designed to operate in a liquid of high dielectric constant. The use of a matching liquid can cut each dimension of the antenna by a factor of $1/\sqrt{\varepsilon_r}$, with ε_r being the liquid relative permittivity. Such a technique, however, asks for a supportive substrate that also has a high dielectric constant. This imposes an extra condition on the selection of the coupling liquid that will be discussed later. In the case of AVAs of the proposed system, a 2 mm ceramic layer (T-Ceram, E-37) with a relative permittivity of 37 was utilized for each antenna. **Figure 4** shows the design parameters of an AVA alongside with a photo of a pair of fabricated AVAs. The exponential curves y_a, y_t, and y_f shown in the figure are given by the following Eq. [90]:

$$y_k = \pm\left(A_k e^{P_k(x-B_k)} + C_k\right) \tag{1}$$

where

$$A_k = \frac{y_{k1} - y_{k2}}{e^{P_k(x_{k1}-B_k)} - e^{P_k(x_{k2}-B_k)}},\ C_k = \frac{y_{k1}e^{P_i x_{k2}} - y_{k2}e^{P_k x_{k1}}}{e^{P_k x_{k2}} - e^{P_k x_{k1}}} \tag{2}$$

and k can be substituted with a, t, or f to obtain y_a, y_t, or y_f, in order. The subscripts 1 and 2 for x denote the x-coordinate of the start point and endpoint of the curves. The constants A_i, B_i, C_i, and P_i for every equation are given in **Table 1**. The numerical values of the parameters for the

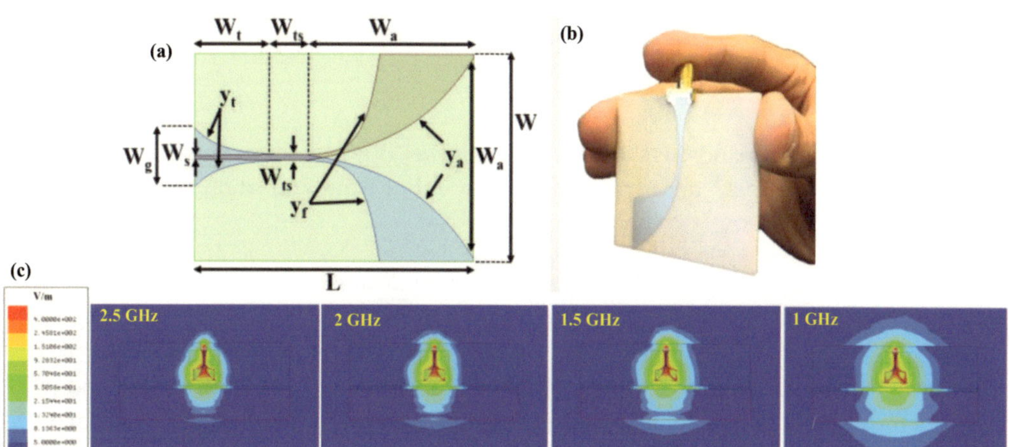

Figure 4. (a) Design parameters of the AVA used in the system. This transparent view of the antenna shows the curves on front (signal) and back (ground) of the antenna. (b) The fabricated antenna has a reduced size, as it can be seen when the size is compared to a person's hand. (c) The simulated results showing the magnitude of the electric field inside an ethanol model at different frequencies.

$y_i(x)$	A	B	C	P
y_t	$\frac{W_{ts}-W_g}{2(e^{P_t L_t}-1)}$	0	$\frac{W_g}{2}-A_t$	P_t
y_f	A_f	W_t+W_{ts}	$\frac{W_{ts}}{2}-A_f$	P_f
y_a	$\frac{W_{ts}+W_a}{2(e^{P_a L_a}-1)}$	W_t+W_{ts}	$-\frac{W_{ts}}{2}-A_f$	P_a

Table 1. The definitions of the parameters A, B, C, and P in the curve equations of the AVA.

fabricated antennas were $W = 30$, $W_g = 2.06$, $W_a = 25.42$, $W_{ts} = 0.29$, $W_s = 0.025$, $L_t = 8.40$, $L_{ts} = 1.03$, $L_a = 26.54$, all in millimetres, and $P_t = -1.04$, $P_f = 0.94$, $P_a = 0.1$ [91]. The radiation pattern of a single antenna is illustrated in **Figure 4 (c)** at different frequencies.

To select the coupling liquid, the dielectric relaxation of many liquids, such as [92–102], were considered. John D. et al. used multi-step techniques to approximate the average dielectric properties of the breast tissue and reported a minimum and maximum of about 26.5 and 27 for the relative permittivity in 1–3 GHz, respectively [103]. For a proper coupling of the electromagnetic waves, the average dielectric constant of the sought liquid must be between the relative permittivity of the antenna substrate (37) and that of the average breast (26.75). Based on this criterion and other conditions such as non-toxicity, non-carcinogenicity, low viscosity, and stability at room temperature, among many candidates, ethanol was selected as the matching liquid. The characterization of an array of two AVAs in ethanol can be found in [104].

5.2. Radiation safety: Specific absorption rate (SAR)

To assure that the microwave radiation from the antennas was safe for human use, a specific absorption rate (SAR) analysis was conducted. The SAR determines the amount of power absorbed by the human tissue when it is exposed to the electromagnetic radiation [105]. The local SAR at a certain point inside the tissue is defined as

$$SAR_{local}(\mathbf{r},\omega) = \frac{\sigma(\mathbf{r},\omega)|E(\mathbf{r},\omega)|^2}{2\rho(\mathbf{r})} \tag{3}$$

where $\mathbf{r}$ is the position vector, ω is the frequency in $[rad/s]$, $\sigma(\mathbf{r},\omega)$ is the material conductivity in $[S/m]$, and $\rho(\mathbf{r})$ is the mass density of the dielectric. For standardization purposes, SAR is averaged over a small sample volume as follows:

$$SAR_{average}(\mathbf{r},\omega) = \frac{1}{V}\int \frac{\sigma(\mathbf{r},\omega)|E(\mathbf{r},\omega)|^2}{\rho(\mathbf{r})} d\mathbf{r} \tag{4}$$

This power flow reveals itself in the form of temperature gradient over time, and it could cause harm if it trespasses a certain value. Federal Communications Commission (FCC) in the United States has set a threshold of 1.6 W/kg for the maximum value of SAR in a 1-gram sample of body parts [105]. In Europe, as set by The Council of the European Union (CEU), the limit is 2 W/kg in a 10-gram sample of body parts [107]. IEEE Standard 1528 presents a methodology to compute the peak SAR in the head under exposure to radio frequency radiation [108, 109].

http://dx.doi.org/10.5772/intechopen.69726

This can also be applied in other body part calculations. HFSS ANSYS, which automatically applies IEEE standard P1528.4 to calculate the spatial average of SAR [111], was utilized to analyze the SAR of the heat that an AVA induces in a breast model placed directly underneath it. The model consisted of fat distribution data from a real healthy breast, obtained by the DBT system at the Massachusetts General Hospital (MGH). **Figure 5 (a)–(c)** illustrates the fat distribution in the model from different views. In lieu of importing the entire data set into the HFSS, the fat percentage values were averaged over cubes of 6 mm side to lessen the computational load. Next, the complex relative permittivity of the breast was approximated by a Cole-to-Cole model. The impact of the breast compression paddle and the ethanol container were also accounted for by using a simplified geometry of the NRI system, as shown in **Figure 5 (d)–(e)**. In accordance with the real measurements, the power fed to the antennas

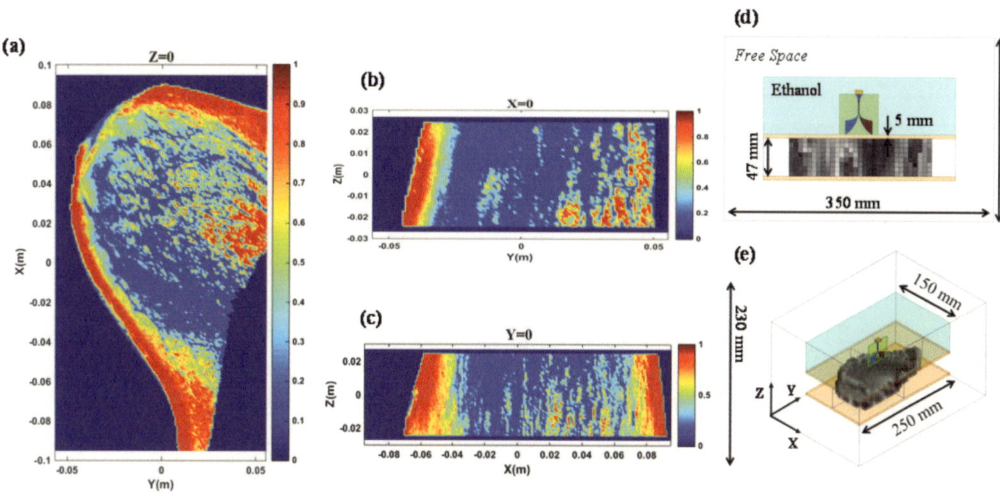

Figure 5. The fat distribution map of a real healthy breast used to compute the complex dielectric constant [106], and its associated model. The map as viewed from (a) top, (b) side, (c) front. The approximated model in a voxel grid of cubes of 6-mm sides, from (d) front and (e) perspective view.

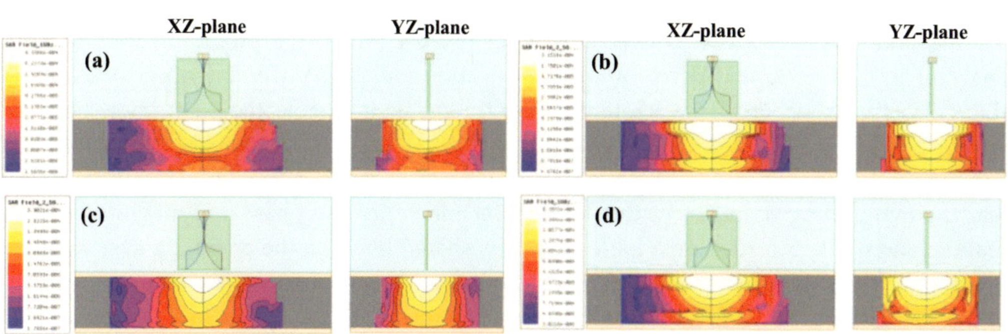

Figure 6. The SAR study results of one antenna radiating towards the breast model: (a) 1-gram sample at 1 GHz, (b) 10-gram sample at 1 GHz, (c) 1-gram sample at 2.5 GHz, (d) 10-gram sample at 2.5 GHz. The maximum value of the SAR occurs at 1 GHz in the 1-gram sample model and is much less than the threshold value set by the FCC.

was set to 0 dBm (1 mW). The results for both 1- and 10-gram sample SAR models at two dissimilar frequencies in the operational bandwidth of the system, 1–3 GHz, are shown in **Figure 6**. As observed, the peak SAR values are clearly below the CEU and FCC thresholds, by at least three orders of magnitude, in all cases. This suggests that the radiation from the transducer array, even with an array of sixteen antennas, is safe for human use.

6. The mechatronic system: Motion stage and data acquisition

6.1. The hardware

As mentioned earlier, to illuminate the entire breast volume under compression, the antennas needed to be moved in a pre-determined trajectory. To accomplish this, a belt-driven mechanical setup was implemented based on the open-source 3D printer, MAKERBOT Replicator. Two motors were used, one for each axis of motion, to enable the planar motion. One of the motors (Y-axis) was fixed to the walls of the container, and the other one (X-axis) was mounted on a carriage that itself moved as the first motor shaft rotated. The dimensions and other geometric properties of the box containing all the mechanical parts were majorly restrained by the compression paddle of General Electric DBT system that was available at the MGH. Given these requirements, two acrylic boxes were built, one on the bottom, serving as the matching liquid container, and one on the top, holding the motion stage assembly in place. Two Big Easy Drivers, powered by a 12 V/5 A power supply, and an Arduino Uno were used to actuate and control the motors. For the bottom box to safely contain the coupling liquid, all of its interior edges were sealed with a silicon-based sealant (General Electric), which was specifically formulated for plastics. Moreover, a lid attached to the top box via hinges was used to constrain ethanol's evaporation. The various parts of the system are shown in **Figure 7**.

6.2. The software

LABVIEW was used as the main programming tool for data acquisition, mechanical motion control, and synchronization between the two. PNA-X (N5242), a programmable network analyzer by Keysight, was used for data acquisition and LABVIEW Interface for Arduino (LIFA) was installed on the workstation (Windows 10) to enable the connection between Aruino and LABVIEW. Using the Stepper Motor Library of LIFA, the motors were configured to have a default speed of 2000 steps/sec in each section of the motion path. The collected data was the two-port s-parameters of the AVAs, which included the phase and magnitude information; and it was recorded on a folder that was shared between the operating system of the PNA-X and the workstation computer. For simplicity, in the first imaging experiments, instead of using triggers to time different events in the acquisition process, a short delay, was utilized after the command was sent to the PNA-X to ascertain that the data collection at each point of the path was complete before moving to the next position. The value of the delay was determined approximately with trial and error. As displayed in **Figure 8**, at any time during the motion on the default path, only one motor is active.

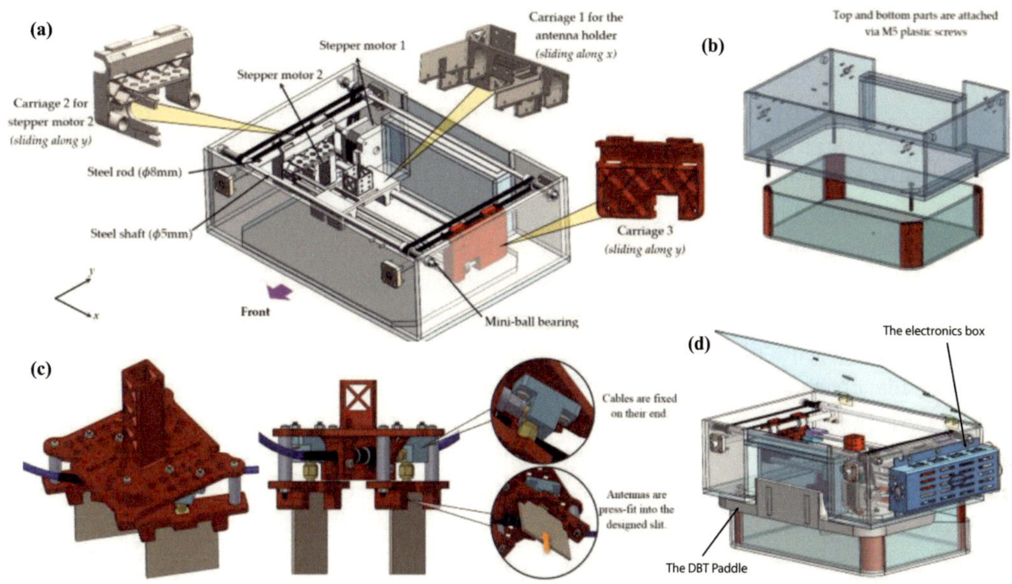

Figure 7. Schematic diagram of the mechanical parts of the motion stage: (a) The gantry on top, responsible for moving the transducer array in two dimensions, (b) the attachment mechanism for the top and bottom boxes, (c) the antenna holder with a structure that assures cables are fixed on the end connected to the antenna, (d) the complete assemblage, including the electronics box, fitted into the DBT paddle.

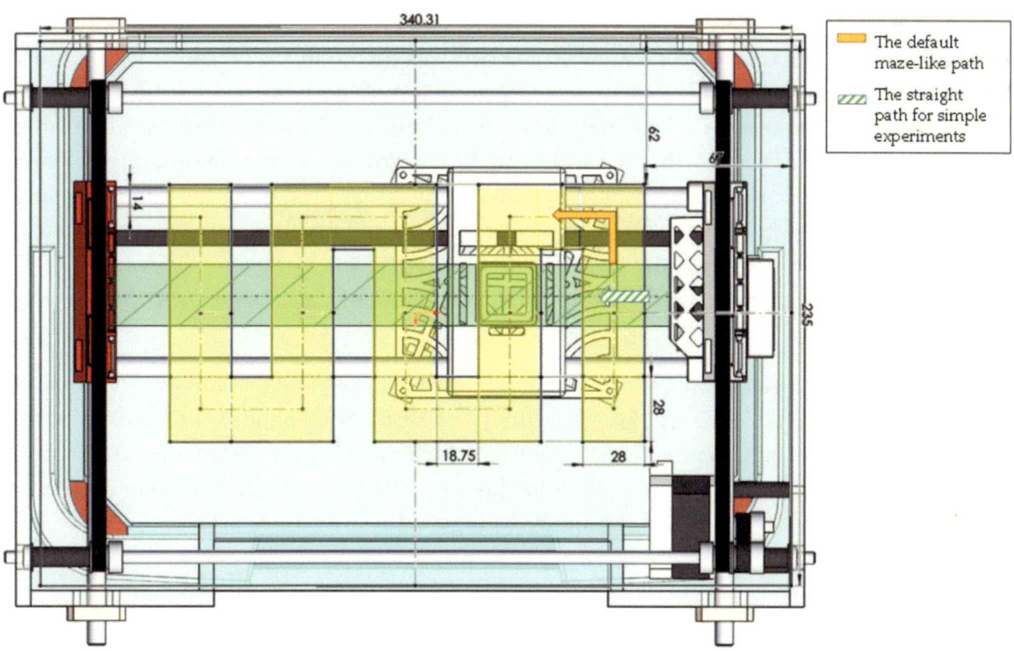

Figure 8. The two-dimensional trajectory viewed from the top. The default path is set to be maze-like (with adjustable number of back-and-forth sections) so that the whole breast volume can be covered. The straight path was used in initial experiments as will be described later.

7. Proof-of-concept experiment and simulation

To show the capabilities of the NRI system as an independent system, a simple measurement was designed to firstly acquire the data from a scattering object inside a known medium, and secondly to retrieve the dialectic map of the medium and the object. This first measurement was simplified using the following requirements: (1) The medium is required to be homogenous with known dielectric properties close to those of breast fat; (2) the object needs to be a strong scatterer of simple and known shape and big size so that it can be easily detected; (3) the data acquisition is to be done in a straight line, instead of the maze-like path, passing through the centroid of the object; (4) the air gap between the NRI system (bottom container) and the under-test medium is to be eliminated. The conditions were realized by using a stainless steel bearing ball of 1-inch diameter inside a container filled with sunflower oil. It is conspicuous that the conditions described differ largely from the reality in which the breast tissue is highly heterogeneous, the contrast between malignant and healthy tissues is comparatively small, and the size of tumors in their early stages is in order of millimeters; however, this first test was intentionally designed to avoid complexities for the purpose of proof-of-concept. Besides this experiment, a simulation was carried out to illustrate how the bimodal imaging using the DBT and the near-field radar system works. The details of this simulation are given in subsection 7.2 and 7.4.

7.1. The bearing ball imaging experiment setup

Required by the imaging algorithm, both the background data, when there was no scatterer in the medium, and the total field data, when the ball was placed in the oil container, had to be acquired. Accordingly, the NRI system was placed on top of the container, partially immersed in the oil, and 25 sets of data at 25 equally spaced positions on the motion path were obtained from the medium with and without the bearing ball inside it. In the case of total field measurements, the ball, seated at the bottom of the container, was positioned at various distances from the centre of the bottom acrylic sheet. The antennas' center motion path was defined to be a straight line passing through the center of the ball, when the system was viewed from the top, as shown with a hashed arrow in **Figure 8**. The layout of the experiment is illustrated in **Figure 9**.

To obtain a more accurate model of the coupling liquid that was used for both the SAR analysis and imaging algorithm, the complex permittivity of absolute ethanol was measured by the PNA-X material measurement software (Keysight Material Measurement Suite 2015), and it was compared against the one reported in the literature [95]. The result is in good agreement with the one reported by Sato et al., as shown in **Figure 10**.

7.2. Imaging algorithm

The total electric field $\boldsymbol{E}(\boldsymbol{r}, \omega)$, assumed to be a function of the vector position $\boldsymbol{r}$ and frequency ω, due to electromagnetic propagation into a three-dimensional medium can be expressed by Helmholtz equation as [111]

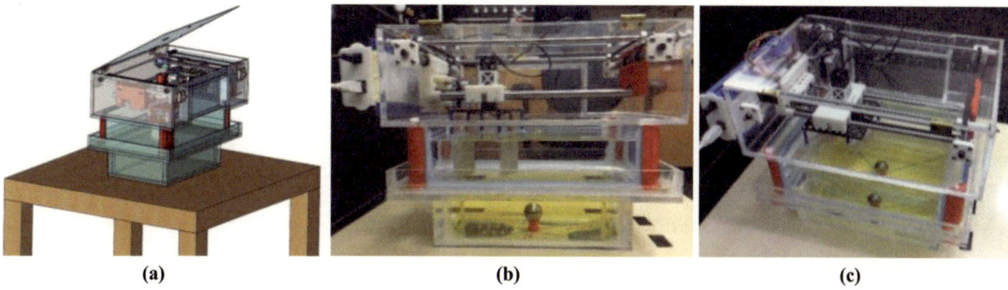

Figure 9. The bearing ball imaging experiment: (a) the entire setup with the NRI system on top of the oil container which is seated on a low-density wooden table. (b) The front and (c) perspective views of the experiment showing how the ethanol container is partially submerged in oil with the aim of air gap elimination. As shown, the ball rests on a plastic base whose diameter is smaller than the ball itself and thus shadowed by the ball when the microwaves illuminate the medium.

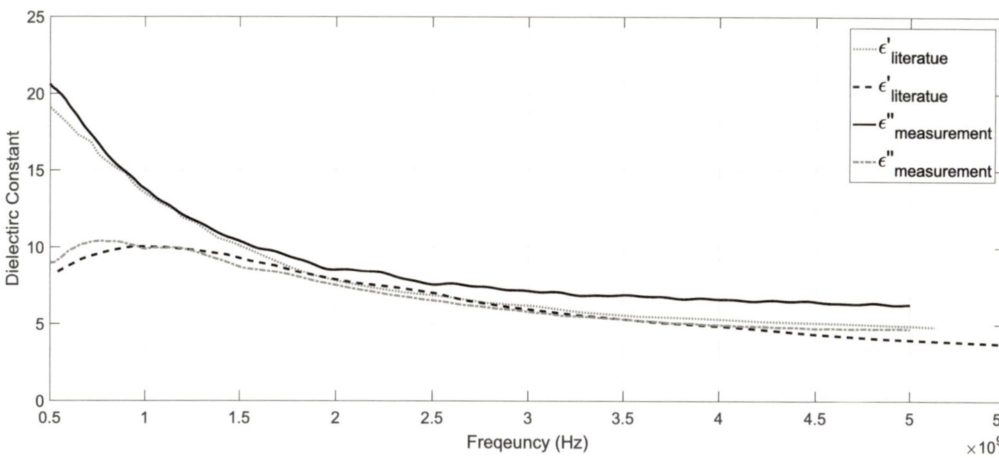

Figure 10. The dielectric relaxation result of ethanol; measurement versus what is reported in the literature [97]. ϵ' and ϵ'' respectively denote the real and imaginary part of complex permittivity.

$$\nabla \times \nabla \boldsymbol{E}(\mathbf{r}, \omega) - k^2(\mathbf{r}, \omega)\boldsymbol{E}(\mathbf{r}, \omega) = j\omega\mu_0 \boldsymbol{I}(\mathbf{r}, \omega) \tag{5}$$

where $k(\mathbf{r}, \omega) = \sqrt{\varepsilon_0 \varepsilon_r \mu_0(\mathbf{r}, \omega)}$ is the wavenumber in the medium with ε_0 being the vacuum permittivity, $\varepsilon_r(\mathbf{r}, \omega)$ being the relative complex permittivity, and μ_0 being the vacuum permeability; and $\boldsymbol{I}(\mathbf{r}, \omega)$ is the microwave excitation source in the case of near-field radar radiation. The relative complex permittivity of a material is defined as $\varepsilon_r = \varepsilon'_r - j\sigma/\omega\varepsilon_0$, where ε'_r is the real part, and $\varepsilon''_r = \sigma/\omega\varepsilon_0$ is the imaginary part that depends on the conductivity of the material σ. The total electric field $\boldsymbol{E}(\mathbf{r}, \omega)$ is composed of the background $\boldsymbol{E}_b(\mathbf{r}, \omega)$ and scattered field $\boldsymbol{E}_s(\mathbf{r}, \omega)$, or mathematically:

$$\boldsymbol{E}(\mathbf{r}, \omega) = \boldsymbol{E}_b(\mathbf{r}, \omega) + \boldsymbol{E}_s(\mathbf{r}, \omega) \tag{6}$$

The background field is usually modeled with the help of simulations or analytical methods, and the scattered field is obtained by subtracting the background field from the measured total field. Since $E_b(r, \omega)$ also satisfies the Helmholtz equation, with $k_b(\mathbf{r}, \omega)$ instead of $k(\mathbf{r}, \omega)$ and the solution

$$\mathbf{E}_b(\mathbf{r}, \omega) = j\omega \int \mathbf{G}_b(\mathbf{r}, \mathbf{r}', \omega) I(\mathbf{r}', \omega) d\mathbf{r}' \tag{7}$$

where $G_b(r, r', \omega)$ is dyadic Green's function and a solution of

$$\nabla \times \nabla \mathbf{G}_b(\mathbf{r}, \omega) - k_b^2(\mathbf{r}, \omega)\mathbf{G}_b(\mathbf{r}, \omega) = \tilde{\mathbf{I}}\delta(\mathbf{r} - \mathbf{r}') \tag{8}$$

with $\tilde{\mathbf{I}}$ being the unit dyad, the scattered field $\mathbf{E}_s(\mathbf{r}, \omega)$ can be solved as

$$\mathbf{E}_s(\mathbf{r}, \omega) = \int \mathbf{G}_b(\mathbf{r}, \mathbf{r}', \omega) k_b^2(\mathbf{r}', \omega)\mathbf{E}(\mathbf{r}, \omega)\chi(\mathbf{r}', \omega) d\mathbf{r}' \tag{9}$$

in which is $\chi = (\varepsilon_r(\mathbf{r}, \omega) - \varepsilon_{r,b}(\mathbf{r}, \omega))/\varepsilon_{r,b}(\mathbf{r}, \omega)$, the contrast parameter, and $\varepsilon_{r,b}(\mathbf{r}, \omega)$ is the relative permittivity of the background medium. In cases where the contrast parameter is comparatively small, BORN approximation can be applied by replacing the total field with the background field in Eq. (9), which results in

$$\mathbf{E}_s(\mathbf{r}, \omega) \approx \int \mathbf{G}_b(\mathbf{r}, \mathbf{r}', \omega) k_b^2(\mathbf{r}', \omega)\mathbf{E}_b(\mathbf{r}, \omega)\chi(\mathbf{r}', \omega) d\mathbf{r}' \tag{10}$$

that can be solved now. Making use of the FDFD method and discretization, Eq. (10) can be linearized in terms of the unknown–the contrast parameter– as follows [112]:

$$\mathbf{y} = \mathbf{A}\chi + \mathbf{e} \tag{11}$$

where $\mathbf{y} \in \mathbb{C}^M$ is the measurement vector obtained by the receiving antenna, $\mathbf{A} \in \mathbb{C}^{M \times N}$ is the sensing matrix, $\chi \in \mathbb{C}^N$ is the unknown contrast vector, and $\mathbf{e} \in \mathbb{C}^M$ is the modeled noise. The sensing matrix $\mathbf{A}$ is generated by the Green's functions of the background medium. Note that for the DBT-NRI system, the background Green's functions are computed using a full wave model (like HFSS ANSYS) in which the dielectric properties of a healthy heterogeneous breast is derived from the fat content of the DBT image. For the results of the bearing ball experiment, presented in this chapter, the background Green's functions are computed from modeling the mechatronic system without the metallic scatterer (ball), also using HFSS ANSYS. As the number of measurements, M, is much less than the number of unknowns N, a regularization method is to be used to reduce the ill-posedness of the solution. In this case, Tikhonov regularization scheme can be applied, which seeks the solution to the succeeding optimization problem [112]:

$$\min \|\mathbf{A}\chi - \mathbf{y}\|_{\ell_2}^2 + \gamma \|\chi\|_{\ell_p}^p \tag{12}$$

$$\text{Subject to}\begin{cases}\mathbf{Re}\Big(\text{diag}(\varepsilon_b)\mathbf{x}+\varepsilon_b\Big)\geq 1\\ \mathbf{Im}\Big(\text{diag}(\varepsilon_b)\mathbf{x}+\varepsilon_b\Big)\geq 0\end{cases}\tag{13}$$

in which ℓ_p denotes norm-p and γ is the regularization parameter. When this problem is solved using $p = 2$, indicating that the ℓ_2 is used as a regularizer function, a simple closed-form solution is given by the following equation:

$$\chi = (\boldsymbol{A}^H\boldsymbol{A} + \gamma\boldsymbol{I})^{-1}\boldsymbol{A}^H\mathbf{y}\tag{14}$$

where $\boldsymbol{A}^H$ is the Hermitian of matrix $\mathbf{A}$ and γ is is selected by trial and error with the aim of achieving an efficient and smooth solution. Other convex optimization approaches can also be used. Specifically, when the problem is solved using $p = 1$, indicating the use of the ℓ_1 as a regularizer function, sparsity can be imposed to the solution—see for example [111]. This regularizer function is of special interest when the DBT and the NRI are operating together.

7.3. Results

7.3.1. Images reconstructed from computational simulations

To demonstrate the efficacy of the hybrid bimodal DBT/NRI system, the fat percentage of the DBT image of a breast was used to model the electromagnetic scattering of a breast with and without a cancer lesion. **Figure 11(a)** shows the ground truth model. A total of six antennas at three different frequencies, 500, 600, and 700 MHz, were used on the periphery of the breast model, inside a bolus liquid, that enhanced the electromagnetic coupling into the tissue [110]. The method described in [106], which used the ℓ_1 norm as a regularizer function, was employed to estimate the real and imaginary parts of the contrast variable χ. As shown in **Figure 11(b)**, the contrast source variable successfully localized the tumor, albeit of being surrounded by fibroglandular tissue.

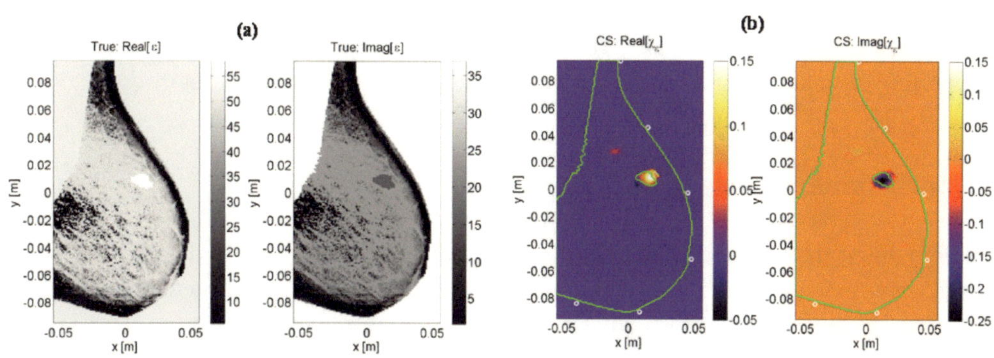

Figure 11. (a) The ground truth complex permittivity, the real (left) and the imaginary (right) part. (b) Successfully reconstructed contrast source variable χ, as defined in Eq. (9), after using the imaging technique described in [106]; (left) real and (right) imaginary parts.

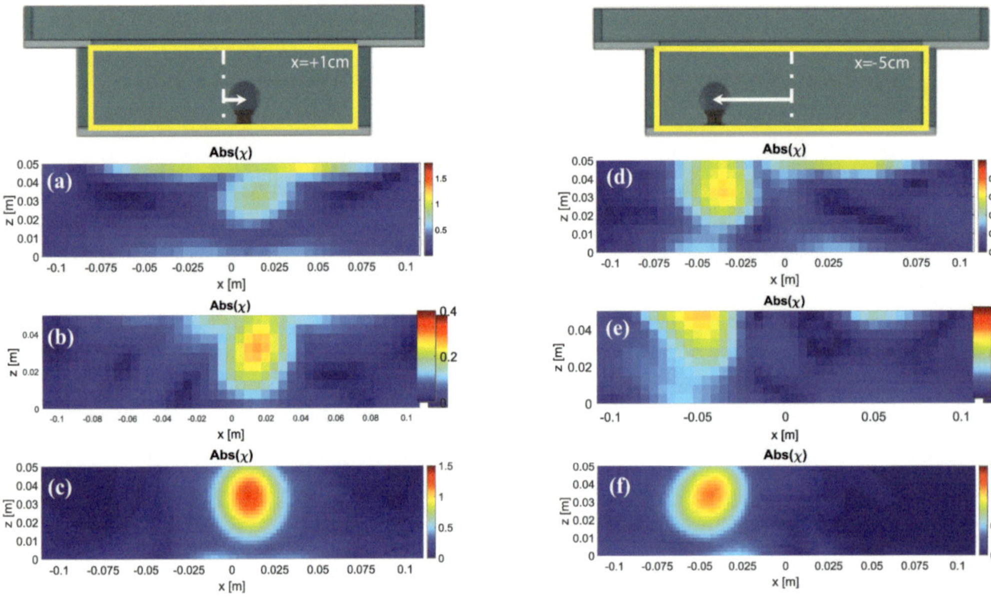

Figure 12. Reconstructed images of a bearing ball embedded in sunflower oil. Images obtained from the data acquired by a regular SMA cable (a), a phase-stable cable (b), and simulation (c), respectively, when the ball was located 1 cm off center. Parts (d)–(f) show similar images for when the ball was 5 cm off center.

7.3.2. Images reconstructed from the experiment

Implementing the imaging algorithm described in the previous subsection, the images of the oil-bearing ball medium were reconstructed for different cases when the ℓ_2 norm is used as the regularizer. As shown in **Figure 12**, the measurements were carried out for various ball locations (two of which are shown here) and for two type of cables, regular SMA cable and phase-stable cable. Despite the presence of some artifacts, the normalized dielectric maps from the measurements agree well with those obtained from the simulations. In overall, though phase-stable cables improved the phase response of the system significantly, they were not as effective in the final imaging results. These images demonstrate that the NRI system is capable of collecting meaningful data and generating images for a simply configured medium.

8. Conclusions

In this chapter, the basics of a bimodal imaging system aimed at early detection of breast cancer were reviewed and some preliminary computational and experimental results were presented. It was noted that the conventional mammography has raised some concerns due to the reported rates of false-positive and false-negative results, as well as overdiagnosis. Digital breast tomosynthesis has been able to compensate for some of these problems, only up to a certain degree, by enabling multi-layer imaging of the breast; and it has resulted in improved specificity and sensitivity. However, the low contrast between malignant and fibroglandular tissues in the X-ray frequencies still remains as a drawback of X-ray-based

http://dx.doi.org/10.5772/intechopen.69726

breast screening. Near-field radar imaging (NRI), as a cheap and safe modality, has the potential to alleviate the problem of low contrast inasmuch as the aforementioned tissues show more contrast at microwave frequencies. Founded on this observation, an NRI mechatronic system, compatible with the DBT, was developed to be used as an auxiliary diagnosis tool, in a co-registered manner. The performance of the NRI component of this system was experimentally evaluated in a near-ideal case, and the achieved results showed its capability in imaging a strong scatterer in a homogenous medium. Computational results were also carried out, showing the efficacy of the bimodal system to detect tumors surrounded by fibroglandular tissue. It was also shown, through specific absorption rate analysis, that the radiation of the implemented antennas is safe for humans, according to the standards. Our next step in this exciting work is to pilot the hybrid DBT/NRI system using more realistic phantoms, as well as human patients.

Author details

Ashkan Ghanbarzadeh Dagheyan[2], Ali Molaei[1], Richard Obermeier[1], Aida K. Martinez[3] and Jose Martinez Lorenzo[1,2]*

*Address all correspondence to: j.martinez-lorenzo@neu.edu

1 Department of Mechanical Engineering, Northeastern University, Boston, MA, USA

2 Department of Electrical Engineering, Northeastern University, Boston, MA, USA

3 Harvard Vanguard Medical Associates, Wellesley, MA, USA

References

[1] Surveillance, Epidemiology, and End Results (SEER) Program (www.seer.cancer.gov) Research Data (1973–2013), National Cancer Institute, DCCPS, Surveillance Research Program, Surveillance Systems Branch, released April 2016, based on the November 2015 submission

[2] National Program of Cancer Registries (NPCR), Center for Disease Control and Prevention (CDC), Available: https://nccd.cdc.gov/uscs/toptencancers.aspx, (Accessed: 13 May 2016)

[3] Howlader N, Noone AM, Krapcho M, Garshell J, Neyman N, Altekruse SF, Kosary CL, Yu M, Ruhl J, Tatalovich Z, Cho H, Mariotto A, Lewis DR, Chen HS, Feuer EJ, Cronin KA (eds). SEER Cancer Statistics Review. 1975–2010. Bethesda, MD: National Cancer Institute, http://seer.cancer.gov/csr/1975_2010/, based on November 2012 SEER data submission, posted to the SEER web site, April 2013

[4] Sugimura T. et al. Heterocyclic amines: Mutagens/carcinogens produced during cooking of meat and fish. Cancer Science. 2004;**95**(4). :290–299

[5] Puangsombat K, et al. Occurrence of heterocyclic amines in cooked meat products. Meat science. 2012;**90**(3):739–746

[6] Beasley JM, et al. Associations of serum insulin-like growth factor-I and insulin-like growth factor-binding protein 3 levels with biomarker-calibrated protein, dairy product and milk intake in the Women's Health Initiative. British Journal of Nutrition. 2014;**111** (05): 847–853

[7] Casa AJ, et al. Estrogen and insulin-like growth factor-I (IGF-I) independently down-regulate critical repressors of breast cancer growth. Breast Cancer Research and Treatment. 2012;**132**(1):61–73

[8] Torfadottir JE, et al. Milk intake in early life and risk of advanced prostate cancer. American Journal of Epidemiology. 2011;**175**(2):144-153

[9] Tate PL, Bibb R, Larcom LL. Milk stimulates growth of prostate cancer cells in culture. Nutrition and Cancer. 2011;**63**(8):1361–1366

[10] Buehring GC, et al. Exposure to bovine leukemia virus is associated with breast cancer: A case-control study. PloS one. 2015;**10**(9):e0134304

[11] Giovanna, Mesa, et al. Bovine leukemia virus gene segment detected in human breast tissue. Open Journal of Medical Microbiology, 2013;**3**(1):84-90

[12] Torre, Lindsey A., et al. Global cancer statistics, 2012. CA: a cancer journal for clinicians. 2015;**65**(2):87-108

[13] Grant WB. Trends in diet and Alzheimer's disease during the nutrition transition in Japan and developing countries. Journal of Alzheimer's Disease. 2014;**38**(3):611–620

[14] Key TJ, et al. The effect of diet on risk of cancer. The Lancet. 2002;**360**(9336):861–868

[15] McPherson K, Steel CM, and Dixon JM. Breast cancer-epidemiology, risk factors, and genetics. BMJ: British Medical Journal. 2000;**321**(7261):624

[16] Mensah GA. Ischaemic heart disease in Africa. Heart. 2008;**94**(7):836–843

[17] Shaper AG, Jones KW. Serum-cholesterol, diet, and coronary heart-disease in Africans and Asians in Uganda. International Journal of Epidemiology. 2012;**41**(5):1221–1225

[18] Sepehrnia B. et al. Genetic studies of human apolipoproteins. X. The effect of the apolipoprotein E polymorphism on quantitative levels of lipoproteins in Nigerian blacks. American Journal of Human Genetics. 1989;**45**(4):586

[19] American Cancer Society. Breast Cancer Facts & Figures 2013–2014. Atlanta: American Cancer Society. Inc. 2013

[20] Christiansen CL, et al. Predicting the cumulative risk of false-positive mammograms. Journal of the National Cancer Institute. 2000;**92**(20):1657–1666

[21] Castells X, Eduard M, Francesc M. Cumulative false positive recall rate and association with participant related factors in a population based breast cancer screening programme. Journal of Epidemiology and Community Health. 2006;**60**(4):316–321

[22] Hubbard, RA, et al. Cumulative probability of false-positive recall or biopsy recommendation after 10 years of screening mammography: A cohort study. Annals of Internal Medicine. 2011;**155**(8):481–492

[23] Cheng HD, et al. Automated breast cancer detection and classification using ultrasound images: A survey. Pattern Recognition. 2010;**43**(1):299–317

[24] Carril JM. et al. Contribution of 99mTc-MIBI scintimammography to the diagnosis of non-palpable breast lesions in relation to mammographic probability of malignancy. Anticancer Research. 1996;**17**(3B):1677–1681

[25] Gram IT, Lund E, Slenker SE. Quality of life following a false positive mammogram. British Journal of Cancer. 1990;**62**(6):1018

[26] Brewer NT, Salz T, Lillie SE. Systematic review: The long-term effects of false-positive mammograms. Annals of Internal Medicine. 2007;**146**(7):502–510

[27] Witek-Janusek L, Gabram S, Mathews HL. Psychologic stress, reduced NK cell activity, and cytokine dysregulation in women experiencing diagnostic breast biopsy. Psychoneuroendocrinology. 2007;**32**(1):22–35

[28] Brodersen J, Siersma VD. Long-term psychosocial consequences of false-positive screening mammography. The Annals of Family Medicine. 2013;**11**(2):106–115

[29] Kerlikowske K, et al. Effect of age, breast density, and family history on the sensitivity of first screening mammography. Jama. 1996;**276**(1):33–38

[30] Dabbous, FM, et al. Comparison of false-negative probabilities for digital and film mammography within a large health care organization. ASCO Annual Meeting Proceedings. 2014;**32**(15_suppl)

[31] Tilanus-Linthorst M, et al. A BRCA1/2 mutation, high breast density and prominent pushing margins of a tumor independently contribute to a frequent false-negative mammography. International Journal of Cancer. 2002;**102**(1):91–95

[32] Meeson, S., et al. Image features of true positive and false negative cancers in screening mammograms. The British journal of radiology. 2003;**76**(901):13-21

[33] Zackrisson S, et al. Rate of over-diagnosis of breast cancer 15 years after end of Malmö mammographic screening trial: Follow-up study. The BMJ. 2006;**332**(7543):689–692

[34] Zahl P-H, Strand BH, Mæhlen J. Incidence of breast cancer in Norway and Sweden during introduction of nationwide screening: prospective cohort study. The BMJ. 2004;**328**(7445): 921–924

[35] Paci E. et al. Overdiagnosis in screening: Is the increase in breast cancer incidence rates a cause for concern Journal of Medical Screening. 2004;**11**(1):23–27

[36] Jonsson H, Johansson R, Lenner P. Increased incidence of invasive breast cancer after the introduction of service screening with mammography in Sweden. International Journal of Cancer. 2005;**117**(5):842–847

[37] Beckmann, Kerri, et al. Estimates of over-diagnosis of breast cancer due to population-based mammography screening in South Australia after adjustment for lead time effects. Journal of medical screening. 2015;**22**(3)127-135

[38] Puliti D, et al. Overdiagnosis in mammographic screening for breast cancer in Europe: A literature review. Journal of Medical Screening. 2012;**19(**1_suppl):42–56

[39] Cole EB, et al. Diagnostic accuracy of digital mammography in patients with dense breasts who underwent problem-solving mammography: Effects of image processing and lesion type 1. Radiology. 2003;**226**(1):153–160

[40] Baldwin P. Digital breast tomosynthesis. Radiologic Technology. 2009;**81**(1):57-74M

[41] Pisano ED, et al. Diagnostic performance of digital versus film mammography for breast-cancer screening. New England Journal of Medicine. 2005;**353**(17):1773–1783

[42] Park JM, et al. Breast tomosynthesis: Present considerations and future applications 1. Radiographics. 2007;**27**(suppl_1):S231-S240

[43] Teertstra HJ, et al. Breast tomosynthesis in clinical practice: initial results. European Radiology. 2010;**20**(1):16–24

[44] Bernardi, D., et al. Application of breast tomosynthesis in screening: incremental effect on mammography acquisition and reading time. The British journal of radiology. 2012;**85**(1020): e1174-e1178

[45] Gur D, et al. Digital breast tomosynthesis: Observer performance study. American Journal of Roentgenology. 2009;**193**(2):586–591

[46] Houssami N, et al. Breast screening using 2D-mammography or integrating digital breast tomosynthesis (3D-mammography) for single-reading or double-reading–Evidence to guide future screening strategies. European Journal of Cancer. 2014;**50**(10): 1799–1807

[47] Bernardi D, et al. Effect of integrating 3D-mammography (digital breast tomosynthesis) with 2D-mammography on radiologists' true-positive and false-positive detection in a population breast screening trial. European Journal of Cancer. 2014;**50**(7):1232–1238

[48] Svahn TM, Macaskill P, Houssami N. Radiologists' interpretive efficiency and variability in true-and false-positive detection when screen-reading with tomosynthesis (3D-mammography) relative to standard mammography in population screening. The Breast. 2015;**24**(6):687–693

[49] Gilbert, Fiona J., et al. Accuracy of digital breast tomosynthesis for depicting breast cancer subgroups in a UK retrospective reading study (TOMMY trial). Radiology. 2015;**22**(3):697-706

[50] Houssami N, et al. Digital breast tomosynthesis (3D-mammography) screening: A pictorial review of screen-detected cancers and false recalls attributed to tomosynthesis in prospective screening trials. The Breast. 2016;**26**:119–134

[51] Rappaport C, Tivnan M, Kaeli E, Obermeier R, Moore R, Kopans D, Martinez Lorenzo J. Fusing microwave radar imaging with digital breast tomosynthesis for high contrast, high resolution breast cancer detection. Radiological Society of North America. 2014 Scientific Assembly and Annual Meeting, Chicago IL. Available: http://archive.rsna.org/2014/14018670.html [Accessed 17-February-2015]

[52] Meaney PM, et al. A clinical prototype for active microwave imaging of the breast. Microwave Theory and Techniques, IEEE Transactions on. 2000;**48**(11):1841–1853

[53] Lazebnik M, et al. A large-scale study of the ultrawideband microwave dielectric properties of normal, benign and malignant breast tissues obtained from cancer surgeries. Physics in Medicine and Biology. 2007;**52**(20):6093

[54] Halter RJ, et al. The correlation of in vivo and ex vivo tissue dielectric properties to validate electromagnetic breast imaging: initial clinical experience. Physiological Measurement. 2009;**30**(6):S121

[55] Golnabi AH. Computational aspect of tomographic microwave imaging for biomedical applications. DARTMOUTH COLLEGE. ProQuest Dissertations Publishing. 2012. 3544495

[56] Meaney PM, Paulsen KD, Ryan TP. Two-dimensional hybrid element image reconstruction for TM illumination. Antennas and Propagation, IEEE Transactions. 1995;**43**(3):239–247

[57] Li D, Meaney PM, Paulsen KD. Conformal microwave imaging for breast cancer detection. Microwave Theory and Techniques. IEEE Transactions. 2003;**51**(4):1179–1186

[58] David W. et al. Three-dimensional microwave breast imaging: Dispersive dielectric properties estimation using patient-specific basis functions. Medical Imaging, IEEE Transactions. 2009;**28**(7):969–981

[59] Joachimowicz N, Pichot C, Hugonin J-P. Inverse scattering: An iterative numerical method for electromagnetic imaging. Antennas and Propagation, IEEE Transactions. 1991;**39**(12):1742–1753

[60] Franchois A, Pichot C. Microwave imaging-complex permittivity reconstruction with a Levenberg-Marquardt method. Antennas and Propagation. IEEE Transactions. 1997;**45** (2):203–215

[61] Rubk T, et al. Nonlinear microwave imaging for breast-cancer screening using Gauss–Newton's method and the CGLS inversion algorithm. Antennas and Propagation. IEEE Transactions. 2007;**55**(8):2320–2331

[62] Gilmore C, et al. Microwave biomedical data inversion using the finite-difference contrast source inversion method. Antennas and Propagation. IEEE Transactions. 2009;**57** (5):1528–1538

[63] Dong Q, Rappaport CM. Microwave subsurface imaging using direct finite-difference frequency-domain-based inversion. Geoscience and Remote Sensing. IEEE Transactions. 2009;**47**(11):3664–3670

[64] Firoozabadi R, Miller EL. Finite element modeling of electromagnetic scattering for microwave breast cancer detection. Skin. 2010;**15**(40.1):0–74

[65] Meaney PM, et al. Initial clinical experience with microwave breast imaging in women with normal mammography. Academic Radiology. 2007;**14**(2):207–218

[66] Neira LM, Van Veen BD, Hagness SC. Investigation of high-resolution microwave breast imaging using a 3-D inverse scattering algorithm with a variable-strength spatial prior constraint. Radio Science Meeting (Joint with AP-S Symposium). 2015;USNC-URSI. IEEE. 2015

[67] Sun YP, et al. CS based confocal microwave imaging algorithm for breast cancer detection. Technology and Health Care Preprint. 2016:1–9

[68] Baran A, et al. Breast cancer imaging using microwave tomography with radar-derived prior information. Radio Science Meeting (Joint with AP-S Symposium), 2014 USNC-URSI. IEEE. 2014

[69] Golnabi AH, Meaney PM, Paulsen KD. Tomographic microwave imaging with incorporated prior spatial information. Microwave Theory and Techniques. IEEE Transactions. 2013;**61**(5):2129–2136

[70] Golnabi AH, Meaney PM, Paulsen KD. 3D microwave tomography of the breast using prior anatomical information. Medical physics. 2016;**43**(4):1933–1944

[71] Klemm M, et al. Radar-based breast cancer detection using a hemispherical antenna array—experimental results. Antennas and Propagation, IEEE Transactions. 2009;**57** (6):1692–1704

[72] Klemm M, et al. Microwave radar-based breast cancer detection: Imaging in inhomogeneous breast phantoms. Antennas and Wireless Propagation Letters. IEEE. 2009;**8**:1349–1352

[73] Klemm M, et al. Experimental and clinical results of breast cancer detection using UWB microwave radar. Antennas and Propagation Society International Symposium; 2008. AP-S 2008. IEEE. IEEE, 2008

[74] Lai JCY, et al. UWB microwave imaging for breast cancer detection—Experiments with heterogeneous breast phantoms. Progress in Electromagnetics Research M. 2011;**16**:19–29

[75] Lazaro A, Girbau D, Villarino R. Simulated and experimental investigation of microwave imaging using UWB. Progress in Electromagnetics Research. 2009;**94**:263–280

[76] Yu C, et al. Active microwave imaging II: 3-D system prototype and image reconstruction from experimental data. Microwave Theory and Techniques. IEEE Transactions. 2008;**56**(4):991–1000

[77] Henriksson T, et al. Quantitative microwave imaging for breast cancer detection using a planar 2.45 GHz system. Instrumentation and Measurement. IEEE Transactions on. 2010;**59**(10):2691–2699

[78] Franchois A, et al. Quantitative microwave imaging with a 2.45 GHz planar microwave camera. Medical Imaging, IEEE Transactions. 1998;**17**(4):550–561

[79] Bassi M, et al. An integrated microwave imaging radar with planar antennas for breast cancer detection. Microwave Theory and Techniques, IEEE Transactions. 2013;**61**(5):2108–2118

[80] Bond EJ, et al. Microwave imaging via space-time beamforming for early detection of breast cancer. Antennas and Propagation, IEEE Transactions. 2003;**51**(8):1690–1705

[81] Li X, et al. Microwave imaging via space-time beamforming: Experimental investigation of tumor detection in multilayer breast phantoms. Microwave Theory and Techniques, IEEE Transactions. 2004;**52**(8):1856–1865

[82] Eleuterio R, Medina A, Conceicao RC. Initial study with microwave imaging of the axilla to aid breast cancer diagnosis. Radio Science Meeting (Joint with AP-S Symposium). 2014 USNC-URSI. IEEE

[83] Grzegorczyk TM, Meaney PM, Paulsen KD. Microwave tomographic imaging for breast cancer chemotherapy monitoring. Antennas and Propagation (EuCAP), 2014 8th European Conference. IEEE; 2014

[84] Fu L, et al. Microwave radar imaging using a solid state spintronic microwave sensor. Applied Physics Letters. 2014;**105**(12):122406

[85] Bucci OM, et al. Characterization of a laboratory setup for assessing the feasibility of magnetic nanoparticles enhanced microwave imaging. Submitted to EuCAP. 2016

[86] Golnabi AH. Computational Aspect of Tomographic Microwave Imaging for Biomedical Applications. Order No. 3544495 Dartmouth College, 2012. Ann Arbor: ProQuest. Web. 13 Nov. 2016

[87] Fang Q, et al. Combined optical imaging and mammography of the healthy breast: Optical contrast derived from breast structure and compression. Medical Imaging, IEEE Transactions on. 2009;**28**(1):30–42

[88] Jiang H, et al. Ultrasound-guided microwave imaging of breast cancer: Tissue phantom and pilot clinical experiments. Medical Physics. 2005;**32**(8):2528–2535

[89] Fei P, et al. A miniaturized antipodal Vivaldi antenna with improved radiation characteristics. Antennas and Wireless Propagation Letters. IEEE. 2011;**10**:127–130

[90] Bourqui J, Okoniewski M, Fear EC. Balanced antipodal Vivaldi antenna for breast cancer detection. Antennas and Propagation, 2007. EuCAP 2007. The Second European Conference on. IET, 2007

[91] Molaei A, et al. Miniaturized UWB Antipodal Vivaldi Antenna for a mechatronic breast cancer imaging system. Antennas and Propagation & USNC/URSI National Radio Science Meeting, 2015 IEEE International Symposium on. IEEE. 2015

[92] Buchner R, Hefter GT, May PM. Dielectric relaxation of aqueous NaCl solutions. The Journal of Physical Chemistry A. 1999;**103**(1):1–9

[93] Sato T, Buchner R. Dielectric relaxation processes in ethanol/water mixtures. The Journal of Physical Chemistry A. 2004;**108**(23):5007–5015

[94] Lu Z, et al. Dielectric relaxation in dimethyl sulfoxide/water mixtures studied by microwave dielectric relaxation spectroscopy. The Journal of Physical Chemistry A. 2009;**113**(44):12207–12214

[95] Markarian SA, Gabrielyan LS. Dielectric relaxation study of diethyl sulfoxide/water mixtures. Physics and Chemistry of Liquids. 2009;**47**(3):311–321

[96] Kavala AK. Dielectric relaxation behaviour of glycine in aqueous solution medium in the microwave frequency region. Indian Journal of Engineering and Materials Science. 2008;**15**:196–198

[97] Shinyashiki N, et al. Shape of dielectric relaxation curves of ethylene glycol oligomer–water mixtures. The Journal of Chemical Physics. 1998;**109**(22):9843–9847

[98] Kaatze U. Microwave dielectric properties of liquids. Radiation Physics and Chemistry. 1995;**45**(4):549–566

[99] Barthel J, et al. Dielectric spectra of some common solvents in the microwave region. Water and lower alcohols. Chemical Physics Letters. 1990;**165**(4):369–373

[100] Saar D, et al. Ultrasonic and microwave dielectric relaxation of liquid dialkyl carbonates. The Journal of Physical Chemistry. 1978;**82**(23):2531–2535

[101] Undre PB, et al. Dielectric relaxation in ethylene glycol-dimethyl sulfoxide mixtures as a function of composition and temperature. Journal of the Korean Chemical Society. 2012;**56**(4):416–423

[102] Bindu GN, et al. Dielectric studies of corn syrup for applications in microwave breast imaging. Progress In Electromagnetics Research. 2006;**59**:175–186

[103] Garrett JD, Fear EC. Average dielectric property analysis of complex breast tissue with microwave transmission measurements. Sensors. 2015;**15**(1):1199–1216

[104] Dagheyan AG, et al. Characterization of two antipodal Vivaldi antennas for breast cancer near-field radar imaging. Antennas and Propagation (APSURSI), 2016 IEEE International Symposium on. IEEE. 2016

[105] Evaluating Compliance with FCC Guidelines for Human Exposure to Radiofrequency Electromagnetic Fields. OET Bulletin 65, Edition 97-01, August 1997. Accessed at: https://transition.fcc.gov/Bureaus/Engineering_Technology/Documents/bulletins/oet65/oet65.pdf, 13 April, 2016

[106] Martinez-Lorenzo JA, Basukoski A, Quivira F, Rappaport C, Moore R, Kopans D. Composite models for microwave dielectric constant characterization of breast tissues. CD Proceedings. AP-S 2013—IEEE AP-S International Symposium, Orlando, FL, Jul. 2013

[107] The Council Of The European Union, Implementation report on the Council Recommendation limiting the public exposure to electromagnetic fields (0 Hz to 300 GHz), Accessed at http://ec.europa.eu/health/ph_determinants/environment/EMF/implement_rep_en.pdf, 14 April, 2016

[108] IEEE Recommended Practice for Determining the Peak Spatial-Average Specific Absorption Rate (SAR) in the Human Head from Wireless Communications Devices: Measurement Techniques - Redline. IEEE Xplore. IEEE International Committee on Electromagnetic Safety, 22 Jan. 2014. Accessed at http://ieeexplore.ieee.org/stamp/stamp.jsp?tp=&arnumber=6719585, 14 April, 2016

[109] Tan Desmond. Modeling the Specific Absorption Rate Distribution of a Smartphone. 2012 ANSYS Inc. Accessed at: http://resource.ansys.com/staticassets/ANSYS/staticassets/resourcelibrary/techbrief/ab-modeling-specific-absorption-rate-smartphone.pdf, 14 April, 2016

[110] Obermeier R, et al. Imaging breast cancer in a hybrid DBT/NRI system using compressive sensing. Antennas and Propagation & USNC/URSI National Radio Science Meeting; 2015 IEEE International Symposium on. IEEE, 2015

[111] Obermeier R, Martinez-Lorenzo JA. A compressive sensing approach for enhancing breast cancer detection using a hybrid DBT/NRI configuration. Journal of Electromagnetic Waves and Applications. Nov. 2016, doi: 10.1080/09205071.2016.1260064.

[112] Dagheyan AG, et al. Preliminary imaging results and SAR analysis of a microwave imaging system for early breast cancer detection. Engineering in Medicine and Biology Society (EMBC). 2016 IEEE 38th Annual International Conference of the. IEEE; 2016

Chapter 3

Microwave Imaging for Early Breast Cancer Detection

Yoshihiko Kuwahara

Additional information is available at the end of the chapter

http://dx.doi.org/10.5772/intechopen.69562

Abstract

We overview the research trend on microwave imaging for early breast cancer detection. The technologies have two categories: ultra-wide band (UWB) radar that reconstructs the scattering power distribution in the breast and inverse scattering problem that reconstructs the dielectric properties distribution. We have developed a clinical equipment using UWB radar and carried out clinical test 4 years ago. Through the experiments, we concluded that the UWB radar was insufficient for the clinical equipment, because the UWB radar cannot discriminate cancerous tumor and other lesions. Therefore, we have been studying inverse scattering. It is a challenging task to develop an equipment using inverse scattering technologies. We have proposed a microwave mammography that has four features: (1) sensor with breast fixing by absorption, (2) small sensor with multipolarization, (3) image reconstruction program linking the commercial EM simulator, and (4) hybrid imaging method using UWB radar and inverse scattering.

Keywords: early breast cancer detection, microwave imaging, radar, inverse scattering, hybrid imaging

1. Introduction

Early detection and treatment of breast cancer, which has the highest rate of incidence in women, are important. Although X-ray mammography is widely used, it has the disadvantages of X-ray exposure, detection failure owing to low contrast, and pain during inspection. An echograph is a well-established alternative to X-ray mammography. However, the inspection quality of this device depends on the skill of the inspector, and the reproducibility of results is poor [1]. Recently, microwave imaging for breast cancer detection has attracted attention [2]. However, the low contrast between fibroglandular tissue and malignant tissue in the microwave frequency range poses a challenge to many researchers [3].

Breast cancer detection through microwave imaging is broadly grouped into two categories: tomography [4] and ultra-wide bandwidth (UWB) radar [5]. Tomography can reconstruct such organization structures as fatty, fibroglandular, and malignant tissues. However, the electromagnetic analysis including the antennas, supporting structure, and environment must be accurately carried out because measuring error, noise, and modeling error significantly affect the image reconstruction. Moreover, since the calculation load is enormous, it is unsuitable for mass examination. UWB radar cannot reconstruct the organization structure accurately [6]. However, since it is tolerant to measuring error and noise in comparison with tomography, it is easy to manufacture. Furthermore, since the calculation load is small, it is suitable for mass examination.

We have developed multistatic UWB radar for early breast cancer detection. Our equipment features multistatic microwave imaging via space time (MS-MIST) algorithm, which extends the MIST algorithm to multistatic UWB radar [5] and a conformal array, which fixes the breast to the inner shape of a sensor via suction [7]. Through numerical simulations and experiments with phantoms, MS-MIST was confirmed to have high resolution with low artifacts. In addition, our sensor requires neither placement of the breast in a tank filled with a coupling liquid nor measurement of the breast shape. The proposed system has low failure rate of inspection in comparison with the already developed UWB radar [6] because the sensor with suction and fixation restrains the patient from moving and breathing during the scan. Moreover, the inspection time is short because the number of antennas is reduced by MS-MIST with high resolution and low artifact. Hence, it results in small size and low cost. First, we describe the clinical equipment developed and demonstrate the imaging results, including numerical and clinical experiments.

The clinical test results demonstrate that the system can detect cancer that has a clear boundary and is isolated from the fibroglandular tissue. However, if the boundary is irregular or if the tumor is buried under the fibroglandular tissue, the system is unable to correctly reconstruct the shape of the tumor [6]. Therefore, we are currently working on the development of microwave tomography [8–11].

In order to achieve accurate image reconstruction, it is necessary to obtain diverse observation data. Several methods can be employed to obtain diverse observation data. More observation data can be obtained by increasing the number of antennas; however, the scale of the apparatus increases and the computational cost becomes substantial. Furthermore, the signal-to-noise ratio (SNR) is degraded by increasing the size, which degrades the image reconstruction. A method using multiple frequencies has been proposed [12]. In general, biological tissue is a medium with frequency dependence, and its behavior is modeled using the Debye approximation with several parameters. Consequently, the number of unknown parameters increases with the number of frequencies; thus, the reconstruction becomes difficult.

The multiple-polarization method has been examined as a means to obtain a variety of observation data. The impact of polarization on image reconstruction was evaluated in Ref. [13], and it was concluded that the effectiveness was limited. However, the physical considerations related to antenna arrangement have not yet been investigated. Second, we review a compact-sized imaging sensor using multipolarization. We use the distorted Born iterative method (DBIM) described in Ref. [12] to solve the inverse scattering problem.

Microwave tomography can reconstruct complex structures if the measurement system is modeled completely and there is no measurement error. In order to reduce the modeling error, an image-reconstructing program that solves the forward problem using a commercial electromagnetic simulator has been developed [9]. Considering the actual device, this program includes an algorithm that applies the scattering parameters provided by the vector network analyzer (VNA) to the inverse scattering equation [10]. Third, we present microwave mammography with these technologies.

We could successfully reconstruct the complex numerical breast phantom using the proposed microwave mammography. Subsequently, we developed simple microwave tomography and carried out experiments. However, we could not reconstruct a sufficiently high-quality image owing to the deviations between the calculated and measured backscattered signals. It is well known that the settings of the initial complex permittivity distribution are important. Previously, initial permittivity in the imaging area was set to be uniform. Finally, we propose a method in which the backscattered power distribution is reconstructed by the radar, and the distribution is subsequently used as the prior knowledge in the inverse scattering problem. The effectiveness of the proposed method is confirmed by experiments.

2. Breast model and propagation analysis

2.1. Electromagnetic property of the breast

The breast cancer detection based on microwave imaging relies on large differences in the electromagnetic properties between normal and malignant tissues. In quantitative microwave imaging, considering the biological tissues as dielectrics, the dielectric properties are reconstructed according to the differences in the complex permittivity, defined by Eq. (1):

$$\varepsilon^* = \varepsilon_r + j\frac{\sigma}{\omega\varepsilon_0} \tag{1}$$

where ε_r is the relative permittivity, σ is the conductivity of examined object, ε_0 is the free-space permittivity, and ω is the angular frequency.

The electromagnetic properties of breast tissue in different frequency ranges have been studied. Gabriel et al. conducted a major review of measured dielectric properties on healthy human tissues for frequencies between 10 Hz and 100 GHz [14]. In the study, the basic and well-known Debye model in Eq. (2) is introduced:

$$\varepsilon^*(\omega) = \varepsilon_\infty + \frac{\varepsilon_s - \varepsilon_\infty}{1 + j\omega\tau} \tag{2}$$

This equation is extended to the Cole-Cole expression to model the structure and composition of biological tissues, defined in Eq. (3):

$$\varepsilon^*(\omega) = \varepsilon_\infty + \frac{\Delta\varepsilon}{1 + j\omega\tau} + \frac{\sigma_s}{j\omega\varepsilon_0} \tag{3}$$

where ε_∞ is the static frequency permittivity constants, and σ_s is the static conductivity. The magnitude of dispersion is $\Delta\varepsilon = \varepsilon_s - \varepsilon_\infty$. The relaxation time constant τ is assumed to be spatially invariant and usually considered to be in the range of 15–17 ps.

Furthermore, female breast tissues have been studied with focus on breast tumor detection. *Ex vivo* measurements of fresh human malignant and normal breast tissues have been performed by several groups. Lazebnik et al. reported the most comprehensive examination of the dielectric properties of normal, benign, and malignant breast tissues [3].

2.2. Electromagnetic analysis

Microwave mammography consists of multiple antennas placed around the breast as shown in **Figure 1**. An antenna is selected, and subsequently, a microwave signal is transmitted. At this time, the signals received by other antennas are collected. The transmitting antennas are sequentially selected to obtain the received data. We reconstruct the image using a set of received data. In tomography, this physical phenomenon is modeled using a computer. Since the electric constant distribution of the image area is unknown, it is initialized with an appropriate value and repeatedly updated using Newton's method. It is necessary to obtain the electromagnetic field distribution of the image area to apply the Newton's method.

Several methods can be used to solve the electromagnetic problem, including the method of moment (MoM), finite element (FEM), and finite-difference time-domain (FDTD) [15]. It is a very difficult task to prepare the original program using these methods.

In recent years, many commercial electromagnetic field analysis simulators have been developed and widely used for antenna design, electromagnetic compatibility analysis, etc. Commercial simulators are well debugged, and various methods for modeling with high accuracy are adopted. Many simulators have functions to link with external software. We linked

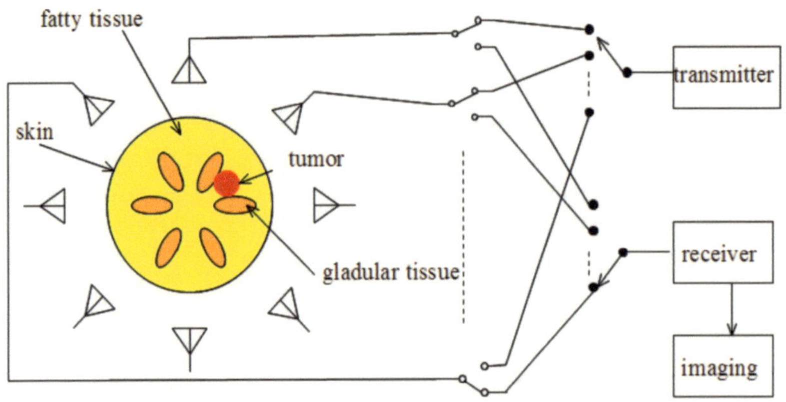

Figure 1. Breast screening by microwave imaging.

MATLAB with simulators such as FEMTET, MW-S, and HFSS, analyzed the electromagnetic field with a simulator, and reconstructed the image using the MATLAB program. If the modeling error is disregarded, electromagnetic field analysis using the FDTD method or MoM is possible.

3. Image reconstruction algorithm

In this section, we overview the image reconstruction algorithm using a microwave signal.

3.1. UWB radar

Ultra-wide band (UWB) radar reconstructs the backscattered power distribution in the breast. The image does not accurately reflect the tissue structure of the breast. However, it may be possible to detect the presence or absence of abnormality such as cancer and its position. Recently, new findings such as adaptive beamforming, utilization of the symmetrical structure of left and right breasts, combined use of magnetic nanoparticles, etc. have been proposed. These proposals can be powerful tools for UWB radar.

3.1.1. Delay and sum

Figure 2 shows the principle of imaging by delay and sum. Consider a scatterer in the imaging area and an array antenna around it. We set a focal point in the imaging area and assume there is a scatterer at that position. When a pulse is transmitted from one antenna and received by the same antenna, the arrival time of the reflected waveform is delayed for the antenna away from the scatterer. Assuming that the distance from the receiving antenna to the transmitting antenna via the focal length is l and the propagation velocity of the wave is v, the time required for the radio waves emitted from the transmitting antenna to arrive at the receiving antenna is $t = l/v$ [s]. When calculating the arrival time required for each antenna and advancing the time response by that amount, if there is a scatterer in the focal point, a coherent time response is obtained and a large response can be obtained by summing. If there are no scatterers in the focus, a large response cannot be obtained even after summing. Subsequently, the focal point is moved within the imaging area, the time response is reversed, and the distribution map is created. The power will be large at the position where the scatterer is present, and it becomes small at the position where the scatterer is absent. This is the same as the imaging principle of the ultrasonic diagnostic apparatus. In this scheme, a narrow pulse with wideband is used to enhance the resolution. Moreover, the algorithm can be easily extended to multistatic radars with different receiving and transmitting antennas.

3.1.2. Microwave imaging via space time

In microwave imaging via space time (MIST) beamforming for wideband monostatic radar [16], the beamformer weights that adjust the array gain at a set focal position in a unit are determined by the least mean square scheme. The transmitting and receiving antennas are identical. In our approach, several receiving antennas are used. Robust and clear images can be expected because

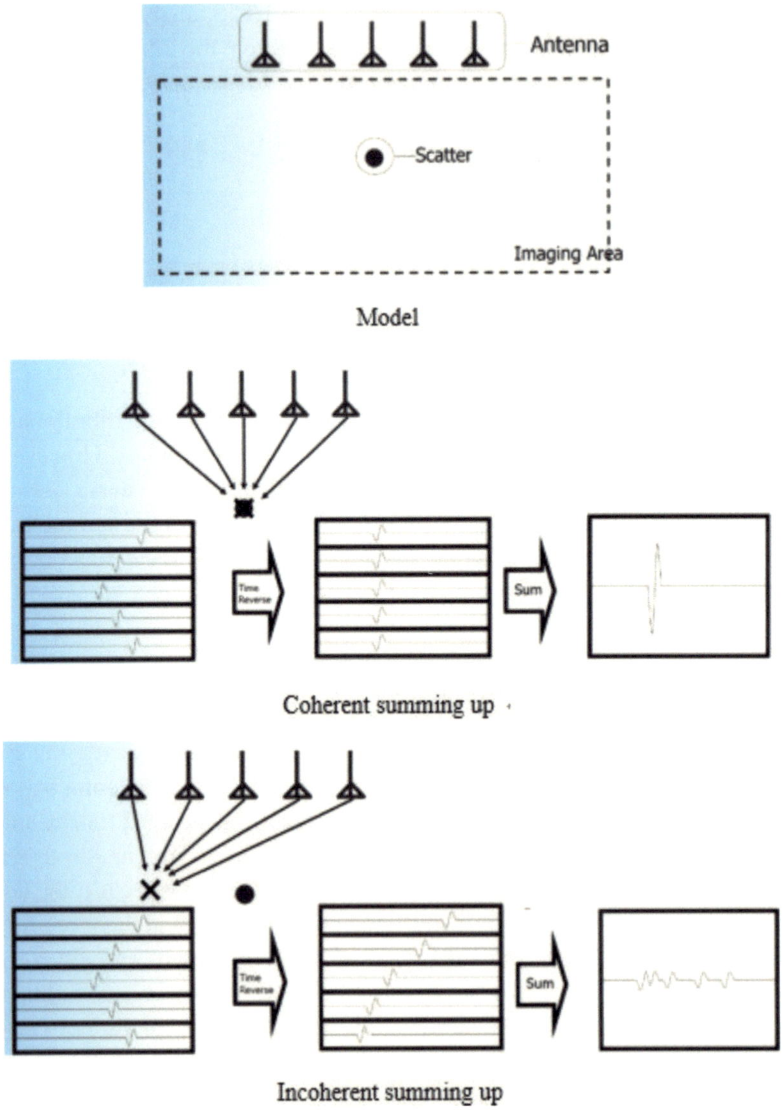

Figure 2. Delay-and-sum.

the scattered response from the tumor enhances the contrast. By computing the output power distribution of the beamformer over the imaging area, a three-dimensional image of backscattered power is reconstructed. The tumor can be detected because a large amount of scattering occurs around it. The weight of the conventional MIST beamformer is expressed by the following formula:

$$W_i(l) = \frac{I(\omega_l)\hat{S}_{ii}(\boldsymbol{r}_0, \omega_l)e^{j\omega_i\tau_0 T_s}}{|I(\omega_l)\hat{S}_{ii}(\boldsymbol{r}_0, \omega_l)|\{1 + |I(\omega_l)|\sum_{i=1}^{M}\hat{S}_{ii}(\boldsymbol{r}_0, \omega_l)\}} \tag{4}$$

where $I(\omega_l)$, $\hat{S}_{ii}(\boldsymbol{r}_0, \omega_l)$, τ_0, T_s, and M denote the spectral component of the transmitting signal at frequency ω_l, monostatic radar response of the ith antenna at position $\boldsymbol{r}_0$, excluding the phase shifts owing to the propagation delays, average propagation delay of the beamformer, sampling period, and number of elements, respectively. The weight of the proposed beamformer is expressed by the following formula:

$$W_{ij}(l) = \frac{I(\omega_l)\hat{S}_{ij}(\boldsymbol{r}_0, \omega_l)e^{j\omega_i\tau_0 T_s}}{|I(\omega_l)\hat{S}_{ij}(\boldsymbol{r}_0, \omega_l)|\{1 + |I(\omega_l)|\sum_{i=1}^{M}\sum_{j=1}^{M}\hat{S}_{ij}(\boldsymbol{r}_0, \omega_l)\}} \tag{5}$$

where $\hat{S}_{ij}(\boldsymbol{r}_0, \omega_l)$ is the multistatic radar response at position $\boldsymbol{r}_0$, excluding the phase shifts owing to the propagation delays when the ith and jth antennas are used as the transmitting and receiving antennas, respectively.

3.2. Inverse scattering (microwave tomography)

3.2.1. Theory

Figure 3 shows the flow of image reconstruction with the inverse scattering problem. First, E^s_{meas}, i.e., the measured data for all the combinations of transmitting and receiving antennas are collected. On the other hand, the contrast based on electric properties is initialized in C_0 in the work station. Based on the current contrast, E^s_{calc}, i.e., calculated data for all the combinations are estimated. Simultaneously, Jacobian, i.e., the sensitivity matrix J is also calculated based on

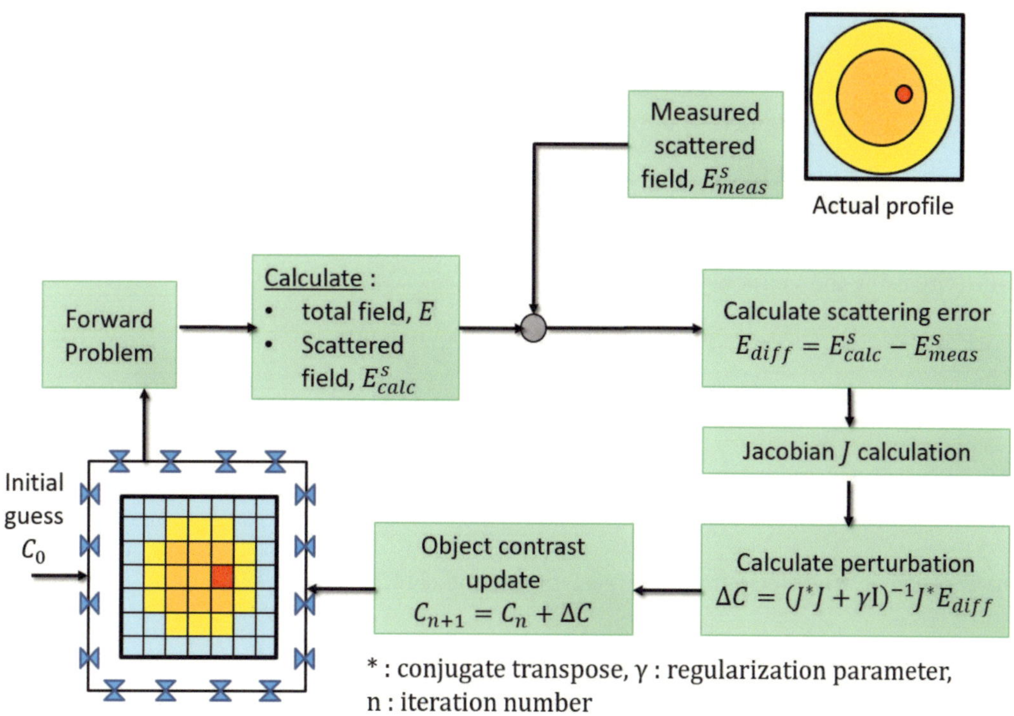

Figure 3. Inverse scattering problem.

the total field in the imaging area E. After calculating perturbation of the contrast ΔC, the contrast is renewed.

3.2.2. Distorted born iterative method

In the DBIM, the relationship between the relative permittivity ε, conductivity σ, and scattering field e^s is expressed as follows [12]

$$\begin{bmatrix} R_e(e^s) \\ I_m(e^s) \end{bmatrix} = \begin{bmatrix} R_e\left\{\frac{\partial F}{\partial \varepsilon}\boldsymbol{B}\frac{\partial F}{\partial \sigma}\boldsymbol{B}\right\} \\ I_m\left\{\frac{\partial F}{\partial \varepsilon}\boldsymbol{B}\frac{\partial F}{\partial \sigma}\boldsymbol{B}\right\} \end{bmatrix} \begin{bmatrix} \varepsilon_1 - \varepsilon_1^b \\ \vdots \\ \varepsilon_K - \varepsilon_K^b \\ \sigma_1 - \sigma_1^b \\ \vdots \\ \sigma_K - \sigma_K^b \end{bmatrix}$$
$$\boldsymbol{B} = \left[\boldsymbol{H}_{1,1}^T \boldsymbol{H}_{1,2}^T \ldots \boldsymbol{H}_{M,N}^T\right]^T \quad \mathrm{F} = \varepsilon + \frac{\sigma}{j\omega\varepsilon_0}$$
$$\boldsymbol{H}_{m,n} = \left[\overline{\boldsymbol{G}^b}(\boldsymbol{r}_n|\boldsymbol{v}_1)\boldsymbol{E}^b(\boldsymbol{v}_1|\boldsymbol{r}_m)\ldots\overline{\boldsymbol{G}^b}(\boldsymbol{r}_n|\boldsymbol{v}_K)\boldsymbol{E}^b(\boldsymbol{v}_K|\boldsymbol{r}_m)\right] \in C^{3\times K}$$
$$m = 1, \ldots, M, \; n = 1, \ldots, N \tag{6}$$

In Eq. (6), $R_e(\cdot)$ and $I_m(\cdot)$ denote the real part and imaginary part, respectively. Further, ε^b and σ^b denote the relative permittivity and conductivity in the background, respectively. K is the number of discretized voxels in the breast region, and M and N are the number of transmitters and receivers, respectively. F is the complex relative permittivity. $\overline{\boldsymbol{G}^b}(\boldsymbol{r}_n|\boldsymbol{v}_k)$ is the dyadic Green's function for the nth receiver at position $\boldsymbol{r}_n$, and the kth voxel at position $\boldsymbol{v}_k$. $\boldsymbol{E}^b(\boldsymbol{v}_k|\boldsymbol{r}_m)$ is the background electric field at v_k when the mth transmitter is used.

Eq. (6) is transformed to the normal equation, and subsequently, Tikhonov regularization is applied, because Eq. (6) is ill posed in general. We solve Eq. (6) and obtain the solutions $\Delta\varepsilon_k = \varepsilon_k - \varepsilon_k^b$ and $\Delta\sigma_k = \sigma_K - \sigma_K^b$. Subsequently, we update the relative permittivity and conductivity using the solutions as follows:

$$\varepsilon_{k+1} = \varepsilon_k + \Delta\varepsilon_k \; \sigma_{k+1} = \sigma_k + \Delta\sigma_k \tag{7}$$

The DBIM iterates the aforementioned procedure until the terminating conditions are satisfied.

4. Development and clinical test of UWB radar

In this section, we demonstrate the development and clinical test of UWB radar.

4.1. System configuration

A schematic diagram and photographs of the developed microwave mammography equipment are shown in **Figure 4**. The equipment comprises a sensor, aspirator, antenna switch, network analyzer, PC for control, and workstation (WS) for data processing.

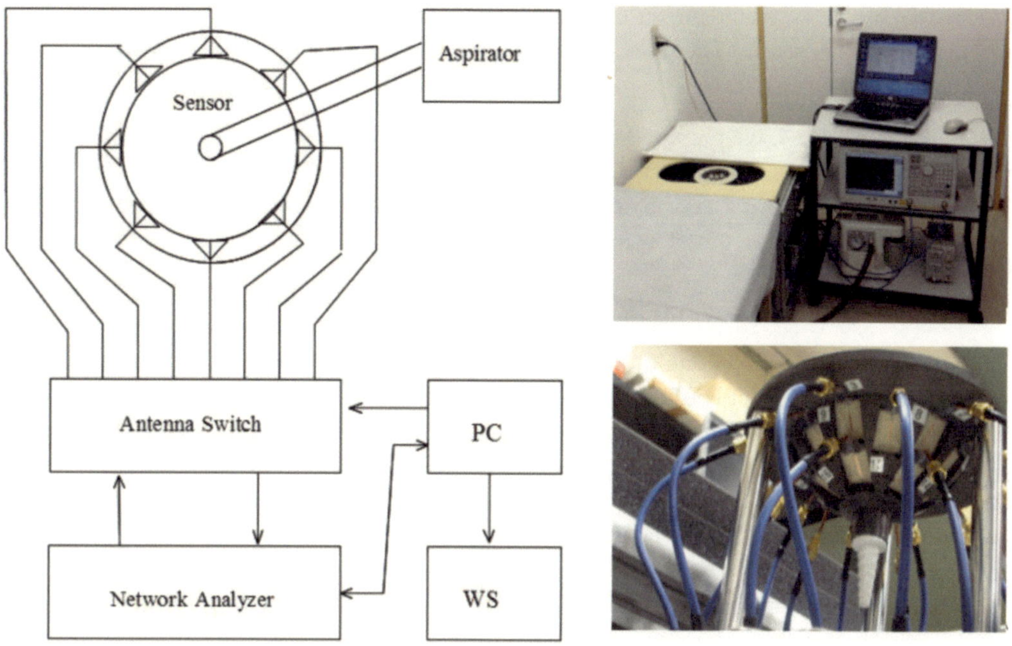

Figure 4. Microwave mammography.

4.2. Sensor

Figure 5 shows the concept of the proposed sensor. It consists of several stacked patch antennas fed by the slot. The number of antennas depends on the breast size. The antennas are embedded in a cup manufactured by Sumitomo Electric Industries, Ltd., whose material has almost the same electromagnetic parameters as the adipose tissue ($\varepsilon_r = 6.3$, $\sigma = 0.15$, at 6 GHz). The elements are designed in order to match impedance over the bandwidth of 4–9 GHz when the aperture

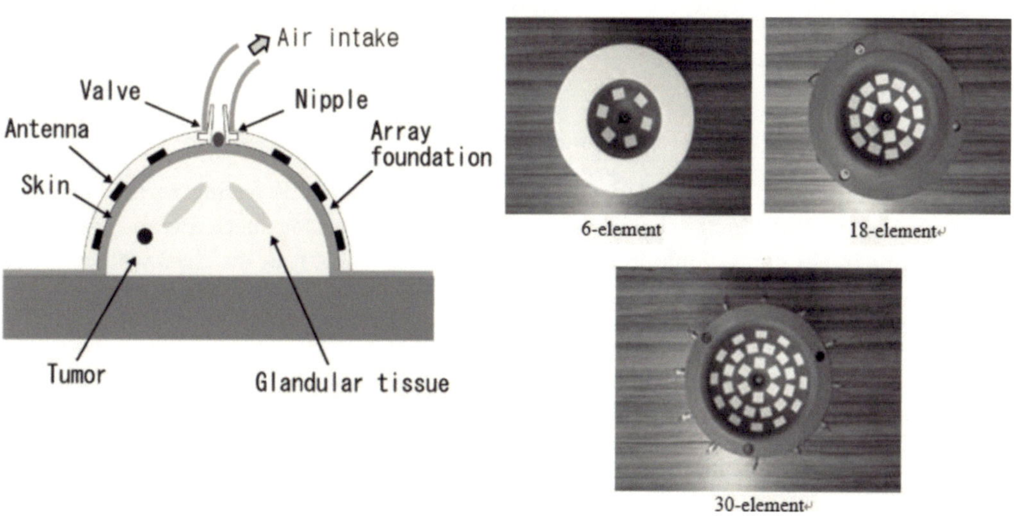

Figure 5. Sensor.

touches the breast. When the pressure in the sensor is reduced by the aspirator, the breast is fixed to the inside of the sensor. Therefore, we need not know the breast shape for the image reconstruction process.

As shown in **Figure 5**, we prepared three different sensor types for various breast sizes: a 30-element sensor with a diameter of 13 cm and a depth of 5.4 cm (large), a 18-element sensor with a diameter of 10 cm and a depth of 4 cm (medium), and a 6-element sensor with a diameter of 8 cm and a depth of 2 cm (small).

4.3. Antenna switch and control

The antenna switch selects one or two antennas connected to the input/output port of the network analyzer (Agilent E5071C) and can correspond with the three sensor types. It consists of 42 single-port double-transfer (SPDT) switches and 6 single-port 6-transfer (SP6T) switches. The total insertion loss is less than 5 dB at 6.5 GHz, and the peak amplitude and phase deviation are less than 0.2 dB and 10°, respectively. The antenna switch and network analyzer are automatically controlled by the PC.

4.4. Clinical inspection

The size of the microwave mammography equipment is 600 (width) × 600 (length) × 500 (height) mm. It is designed to align and connect lengthwise with a bed in the consulting room. Before inspection, a sensor of the proper size must be selected. Using a transparent cup with the same size as the sensor on the breast and subsequently by decompressing, one can confirm that the breast touches all the elements by observation. Subsequently, the patient lies face down on the bed and places her breast in the sensor and suction begins. The value of S_{11} when the breast is placed in the sensor is compared with the value of S_{11} when no breast is present. If S_{11} is not sufficiently reduced, an alarm is activated. In this case, the inspector aligns the position or inclination of the sensor. The inspection time is approximately 5, 30, and 200 s for 6, 18, and 30 sensor elements, respectively. An array rotation technique is used for artifact removal [5]. Additional inspection when the sensor is mechanically rotated by 20° is carried out.

4.5. Imaging results

4.5.1. Early breast cancer in fatty breast tissue

We imaged the breasts of an elderly woman with fatty tissue. Referring to the magnetic resonant imaging (MRI) image shown in **Figure 6**, her right breast is infected with early breast cancer with a tumor that is 9 mm in diameter at the lower inside near the chest wall, whereas no pathological changes can be seen in her left breast. In this case, the boundary of the tumor is comparatively clear, and it is isolated from the fibroglandular tissue.

Figure 6 shows the imaging results using microwave mammography. In this case, a small-sized sensor was used. The reflection strength is normalized by the peak reflection field where it is generated around the cancer. Subsequently, areas where the backscattered energy is more than 80% of the peak scattered power are shown. In addition, the estimated position and size

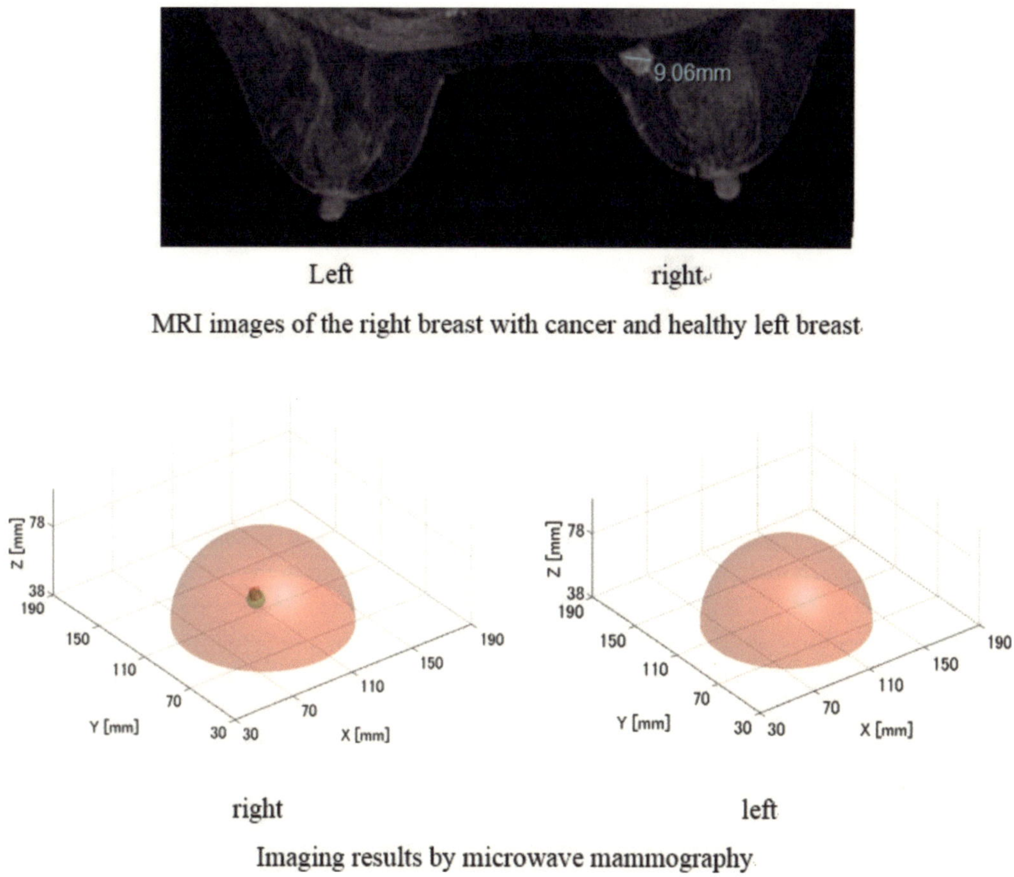

Figure 6. Imaging results: early breast cancer in fatty breast tissue.

from the MRI image are shown with a green circle. These conditions are applied to all the following figures. We can observe a large scattering near the tumor.

4.5.2. Cancerous tumor in rich fibro-glandular tissue

We imaged the breasts of a middle-aged woman with rich fibroglandular tissue. Referring to the MRI Image shown in **Figure 7**, her left breast is infected with a cancerous tumor with a diameter of 1.8 cm at the upper outside near the chest wall. In this case, the boundary is irregular since the cancer is invasive. In addition, it is embedded in the fibroglandular tissue. It is a serious situation for the UWB radar.

Figure 7 shows the imaging results using microwave mammography. In this case, a medium-sized sensor was also used. We can observe a large scattering around the tumor. However, it is difficult to image the outline of the cancerous tumor since the distribution is sparsely dispersive.

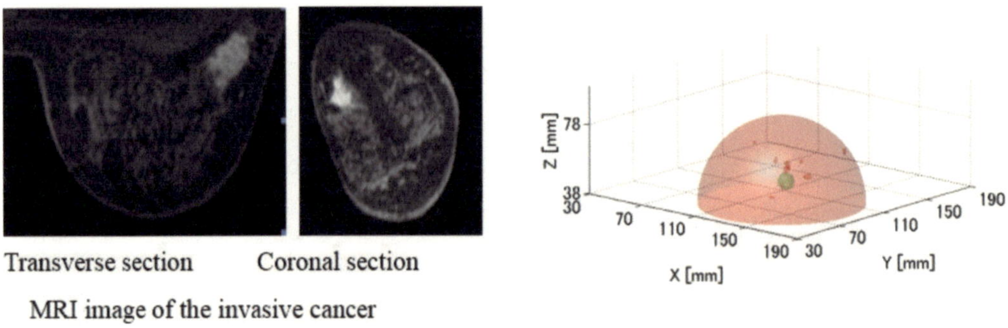

Figure 7. Imaging results: cancerous tumor in rich fibroglandular tissue.

4.6. Discussion

Microwave mammography can detect a cancerous tumor whose boundary is clear and which is isolated from the fibroglandular tissue. On the other hand, it is difficult to detect the cancerous tumor whose boundary is irregular and which is buried in the fibroglandular tissue. In order to overcome the problem, an algorithm to map the complex dielectric constant distribution should be developed by using the inverse scattering problem.

5. Development of microwave tomography

In this section, we describe the key technologies and current status of development of microwave tomography.

5.1. Sensor using multipolarization

In tomography, the breast model is expressed as a set of voxels, and the dielectric properties are estimated in each voxel. The total number of voxels is K, and the dielectric property, which consists of the relative permittivity and conductivity distribution, is represented by the contrast. The calculated data group Y_{mn}, which is based on the estimated model, is compared with the measured data group X_{mn}, which is based on the actual model ($m = 1,\ldots, N$, $n = 1,\ldots, N$, where N is the total number of antennas, m is the number of transmitters, and n is the number of receivers). The contrast (relative permittivity and conductivity) distribution of the breast model is iteratively updated by the DBIM until $X_{mn} \approx Y_{mn}$ is reached.

In the inverse scattering problem, a large amount of diverse observation data is required to achieve accurate image reconstruction with high resolution. In addition, if the measurement error increases owing to low SNR, it cannot reconstruct the image accurately. Therefore, it is better to reduce the analysis region in order to improve the SNR and to reduce the computational cost. When a small sensor is used, a large number of antennas must be arranged in a limited space. In this case, the acquisition of diverse observation data cannot be guaranteed. Subsequently, it is impossible to solve the inverse scattering problem accurately. Nevertheless, various observation data can be obtained even in a small space by changing the plane of polarization.

5.1.1. Simulation model

Figure 8 shows the aperture of the imaging sensor with dimensions 96 mm × 96 mm × 48 mm (width × length × height). The imaging region is discretized into 1183 voxels to obtain 8-mm resolution. A dipole with a length of 20 mm is used for the antennas, and they are arranged in a 4 × 2 configuration on each of the four side panels of the sensor. **Figure 8(a)** shows the position of the antenna. The lines in **Figure 8** represent the polarization direction of the antenna, where the y-axis indicates vertical polarization, and the x- or z-axis indicates horizontal polarization. The antenna arrangements at each side are identical. In this study, we investigated three different configurations as shown in **Figure 8** to examine the effectiveness of polarization in breast cancer detection. **Figure 8(a)** illustrates the vertical polarization, **Figure 8(b)** the horizontal polarization, and **Figure 8(c)** the vertical and horizontal polarization (hereafter referred to as multipolarization).

Antennas are buried in the resin. A hemispheric volume is provided inside the sensor to accommodate the breast model, similar to the imaging sensor with fixed suction proposed in Ref. [7]. The simple breast model shown in **Figure 9** consists of adipose tissues, fibroglandular

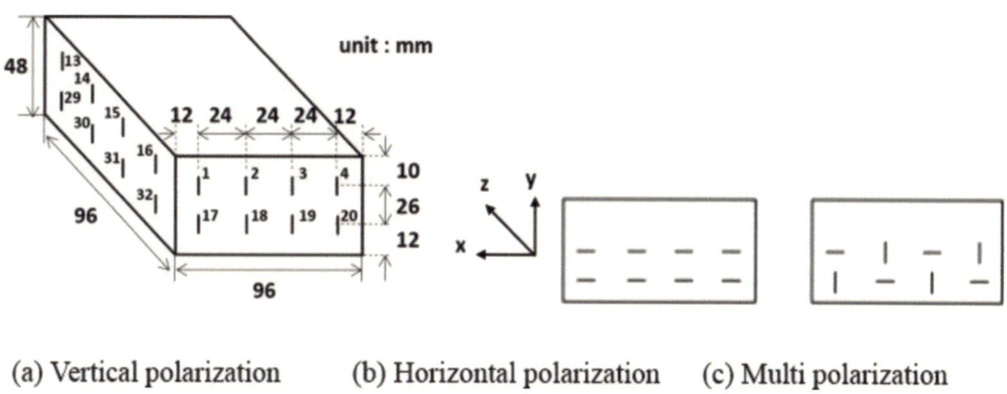

Figure 8. Imaging sensor with various polarizations.

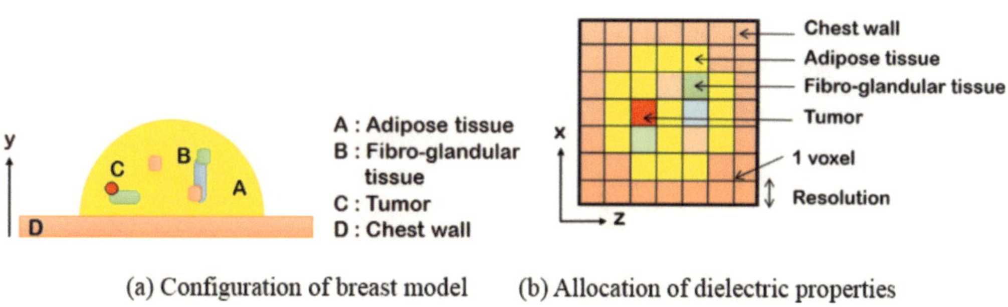

Figure 9. A simple breast model.

	Relative permittivity, ε_r	Conductivity, σ
Background	8	0.15
Chest wall	57	2
Adipose tissue	7	0.4
Fibroglandular tissue	25–10	1–2.2
Tumor	52	4

Table 1. Dielectric properties of breast model.

tissues, and a tumor. The breast model is a hemisphere with a radius of 48 mm, and the tumor has a radius of 4 mm. The chest wall under the breast is also modeled. Ten percent of the volume ratio of the breast is occupied by fibroglandular tissues. This ratio is the average value measured in Japanese women in their 50s. We characterized the dielectric properties of the breast model in each voxel, as shown in **Table 1**.

5.1.2. Numerical results

The total field within the scattering object was calculated according to the method of moment (MOM) as described in Ref. [15, 17]. Further, we used a single frequency of 2.5 GHz. The analysis region consists of the chest wall, adipose tissue, fibroglandular tissue, and a tumor. Moreover, 10% of the volume ratio is occupied by fibroglandular tissues distributed randomly. The vertical and horizontal cross-section of the two unknown parameters, i.e., the relative permittivity and conductivity are shown in **Figure 10**. The units of the x, y, and z coordinates in the figure are meters. The setting model is shown in **Figure 10(a)**, where the chest wall has been omitted. **Figure 10(b)–(d)** shows the results of reconstruction after 350 iterations, using vertical, horizontal, and multipolarization, respectively, for transmitting and receiving data. From the results, we cannot estimate both the relative permittivity and conductivity of the tumor using single polarization, i.e., vertical and horizontal polarization. In contrast, **Figure 10 (d)** clearly indicates the presence of the tumor, and the reconstruction is successful for both parameters using multipolarization.

5.1.3. Discussion

We have confirmed the effectiveness of applying multipolarization to transmitting and receiving antennas in order to determine the dielectric property distributions of a simple breast model. The numerical simulation results demonstrate that the ill-posed problem can be avoided by multipolarization.

5.2. Microwave mammography with a small sensor and a commercial electromagnetic simulator

5.2.1. Imaging sensor with polarization diversity

Based on the discussion in Section 5.1, we propose an imaging sensor with multiple polarizations as shown in **Figure 11**. This sensor is a cuboid, and the aperture size is 96 mm × 96 mm ×

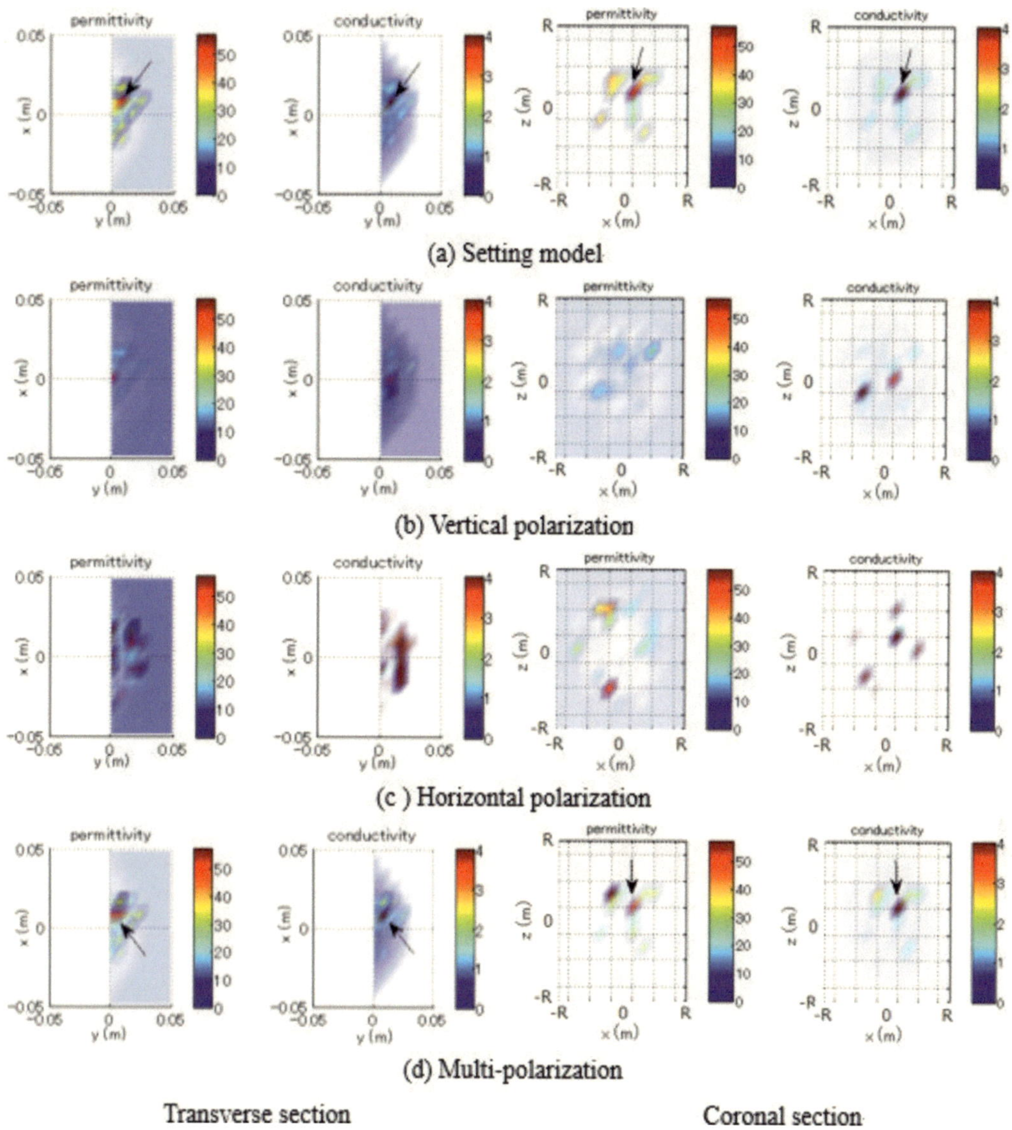

Figure 10. Setting model and reconstructed images after 350 iterations.

48 mm. Six printed dipole antennas are located on each of the four sides, and 12 are located on the top. On each side, the polarization of the antenna changes alternately.

The details of the printed dipole antennas are shown in **Figure 12**. The thickness of the substrate is 0.762 mm, relative permittivity is 10.2, and tan δ is 0.0023. In order to simplify the model, the etching patterns are parallel to either of the *x*, *y*, or *z* axes. The dipole antennas are embedded in the dielectric block whose permittivity and conductivity are almost the same as that of adipose tissue. The resonant frequency is 1.8 GHz.

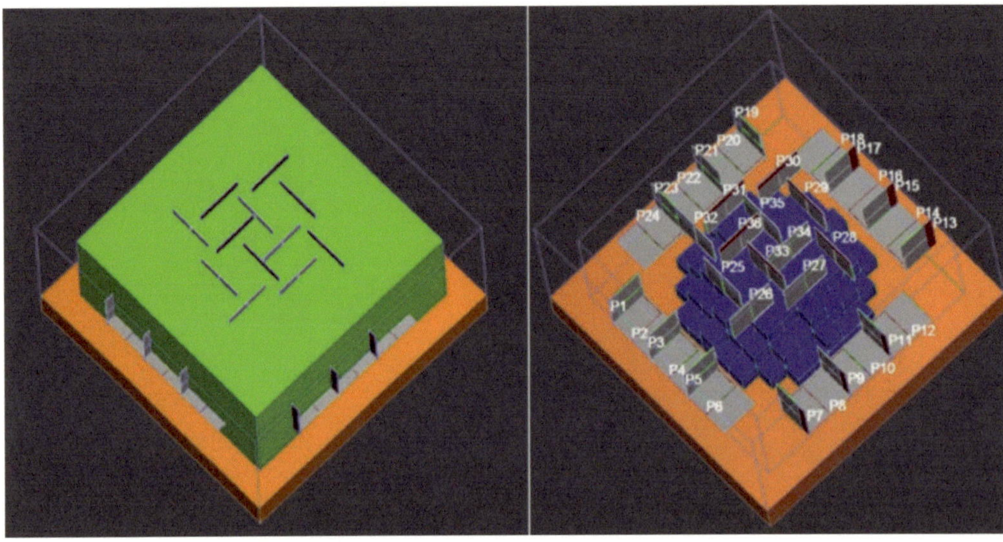

Figure 11. Imaging sensor with polarization diversity.

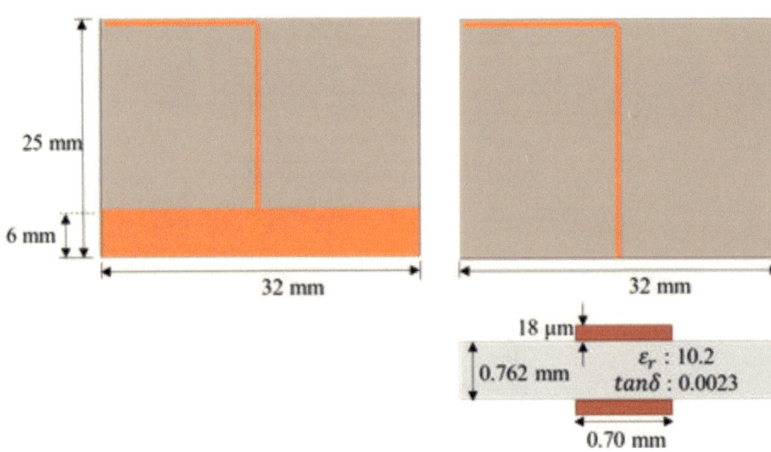

Figure 12. Detail of antenna.

A hemispherical space with a radius of 48 mm and height of 40 mm is prepared for the breast at the bottom of the dielectric block. Furthermore, to absorb the breast, a valve is prepared on the top in order to shape the breast into a hemisphere and to fix the breast to the sensor. With the proposed structure, the breast shape, which is important prior knowledge, can be used in the inverse scattering problems.

5.2.2. Linking with commercial electromagnetic simulator

We can perform electromagnetic analyses with small modeling errors by importing the CAD data of the imaging system into a commercial electromagnetic (EM) simulator. In this study, we utilize FEMTET, which is a 3D-CAE software package by Murata Software Inc. FEMTET implements the finite element method (FEM) and the EM solver can be accelerated by using graphics processing units (GPU). In our image reconstruction algorithm, the procedure of image reconstruction is executed by MATLAB and that of the EM analysis is executed by FEMTET. We can link FEMTET to MATLAB using visual basic (VB) script implemented in Microsoft Excel. The flow chart of the image reconstruction program is shown in **Figure 13**.

5.2.3. *Application of S-parameter*

In Eq. (6), $\boldsymbol{e}^s$ is the difference between the calculated electric field based on the current complex dielectric constant distribution and the measured electric field at each observation point. Since a vector network analyzer (VNA) is used in the actual measurement, the resulting data are the *S* parameter. Since *S* parameters are not directly applicable to Eq. (1), some modifications are required.

On the basis of the reciprocity theorem, the electrical field of the analysis region in the current complex dielectric distribution can be considered as a Green's function $\overline{\boldsymbol{G}^b}(\boldsymbol{r}_n|\boldsymbol{v}_k)$. In FEMTET, it is possible to export electromagnetic fields in a specified region by assuming the input power to the antenna as 1 W. In other words, when $\overline{\boldsymbol{G}^b}(\boldsymbol{r}_n|\boldsymbol{v}_k)$ is given as a field of the analysis region, 1 W can be obtained from the output of the antenna. We consider the image restoration area in a part of the analysis region. While the complex permittivity distribution other than the image reconstruction area is constant, the complex dielectric constant distribution in the image reconstruction area

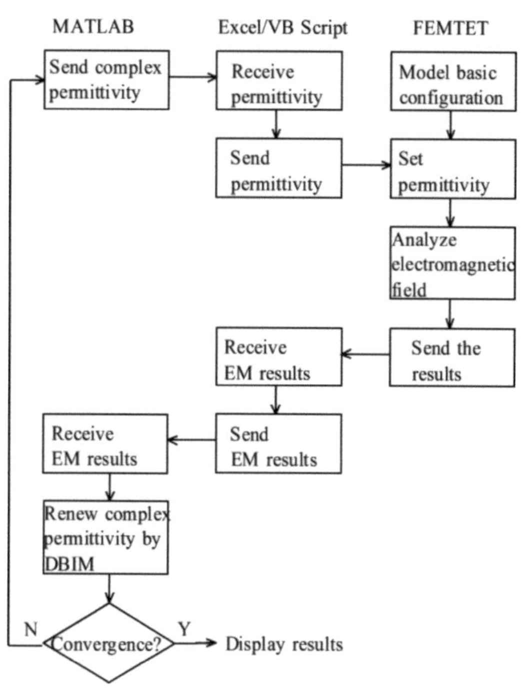

Figure 13. Flowchart of image reconstruction.

is updated. Referring to the structure of the row vector of Eq. (6), the difference between the output power of the antenna before and after the updates can be related to the scattering field on the basis of the change in the complex permittivity distribution of the image restoration area. A sensor including a breast is represented by the multiport circuit network shown in **Figure 14**.

The circuit network equation is expressed using the impedance matrix:

$$\begin{bmatrix} V_1 \\ \vdots \\ V_n \\ \vdots \\ V_N \end{bmatrix} = \begin{bmatrix} Z_{11} & \cdots & Z_{1n} & \cdots & Z_{1N} \\ \vdots & \ddots & \vdots & \ddots & \vdots \\ Z_{n1} & \cdots & Z_{nn} & \cdots & Z_{nN} \\ \vdots & \ddots & \vdots & \ddots & \vdots \\ Z_{N1} & \cdots & Z_{Nn} & \cdots & Z_{NN} \end{bmatrix} \begin{bmatrix} I_1 \\ \vdots \\ I_n \\ \vdots \\ I_N \end{bmatrix} \tag{8}$$

It is assumed that the input and output impedances of the vector network are 50 Ω, and that 50 Ω loads are connected with the antenna ports other than the measurement antenna. When 1 V is applied to the nth antenna, the current flowing in each load can be expressed as

$$\begin{bmatrix} I_1 \\ \vdots \\ I_n \\ \vdots \\ I_N \end{bmatrix} = \begin{bmatrix} Z_{11}+50 & \cdots & Z_{1n} & \cdots & Z_{1N} \\ \vdots & \ddots & \vdots & \ddots & \vdots \\ Z_{n1} & \cdots & Z_{nn}+50 & \cdots & Z_{nN} \\ \vdots & \ddots & \vdots & \ddots & \vdots \\ Z_{N1} & \cdots & Z_{Nn} & \cdots & Z_{NN}+50 \end{bmatrix}^{-1} \begin{bmatrix} 0 \\ \vdots \\ 1(V) \\ \vdots \\ 0 \end{bmatrix} \tag{9}$$

The received voltage V_n can be calculated using I_n (n = 1,..., N). Since 1 W is input to the antenna in FEMTET, the AC power supply voltage is 14.14 V. The Z-parameters can be calculated easily from the S-parameters:

$$Z = Z_0 \frac{I+S}{I-S} \tag{10}$$

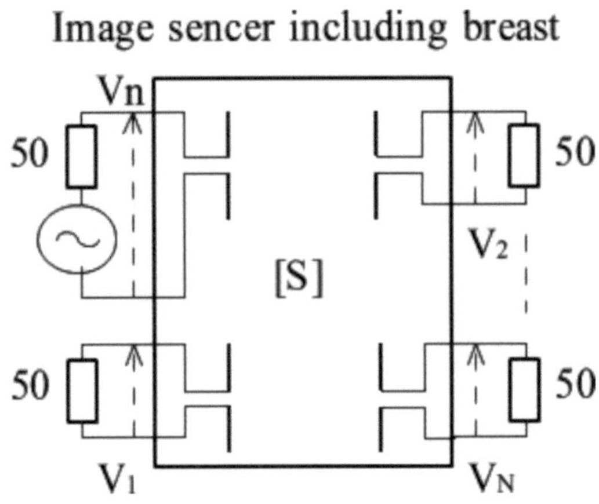

Figure 14. Equivalent circuit of analysis region.

where $Z_0 = 50\ \Omega$, and I is the identity matrix. Applying V_n to the left side of Eq. (6), the updated amount of the complex dielectric constant is determined.

5.3. Numerical test

We have developed a numerical phantom as shown in **Figure 15** on the basis of the MRI image of the patient. **Table 2** shows the relative permittivity and conductivity of each tissue at 1.8 GHz. The permittivity and conductivity of the fibroglandular tissues were set at random within the range of values in the table. The phantom is imported to FEMTET, and forward analysis has been carried out at 1.8 GHz. In the image reconstruction, a coarse mesh was used. The breast region is divided into voxels whose side is 12 mm. Three-dimensional images of the set and reconstructed distributions after 100 iterations are shown in **Figure 16**. In order to quantitatively evaluate the image reconstruction, the reconstructed and set values of the permittivity and conductivity with respect to the voxel number are shown in **Figure 17**. The dielectric constant and conductivity are accurately reconstructed.

5.4. Phantom imaging

We have developed a simple microwave tomography shown in **Figure 18** and carried out experiments. It is made of a dielectric block of size 148 mm × 148 mm × 78 mm with a relative permittivity of 6.2 and conductivity of 0.0367 S/m. Eight dipoles implemented on the dielectric substrate with a relative permittivity of 3.5, tan δ = 0.002, and a thickness of

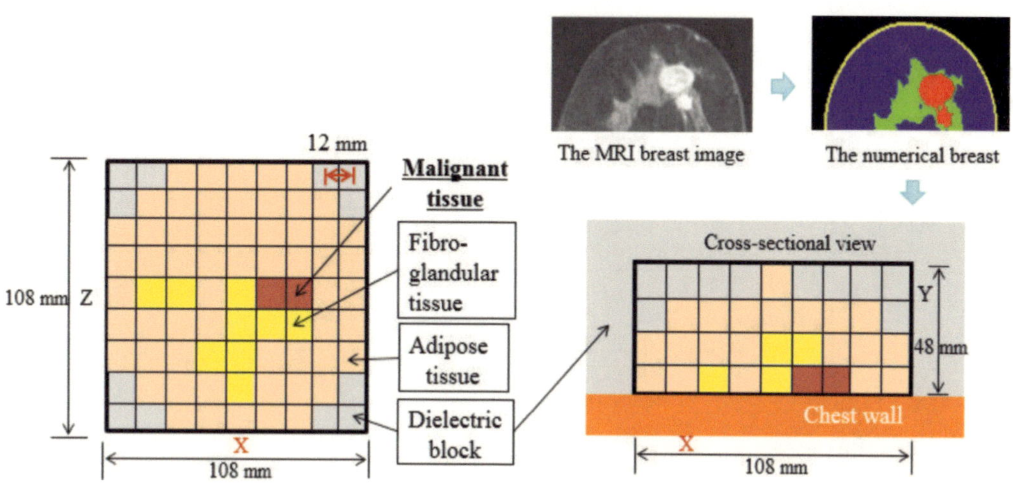

Figure 15. The realistic numerical breast.

	Malignant tissue	Fibroglandular tissue	Adipose tissue	Dielectric block	Chest wall
Relative permittivity ε	52	25–35	7.0	6.2	50
Conductivity σ [S/m]	4.0	1.0–2.2	0.4	0.12	2.0

Table 2. Relative permittivity and conductivity of each tissue at 1.8 GHz.

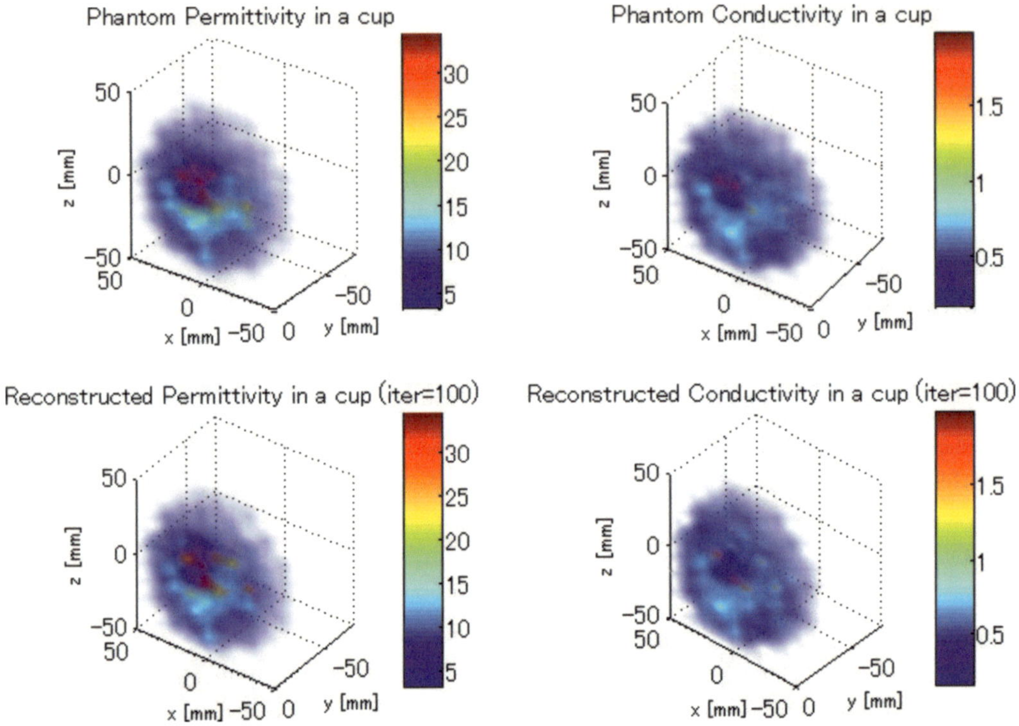

Figure 16. Reconstruction results.

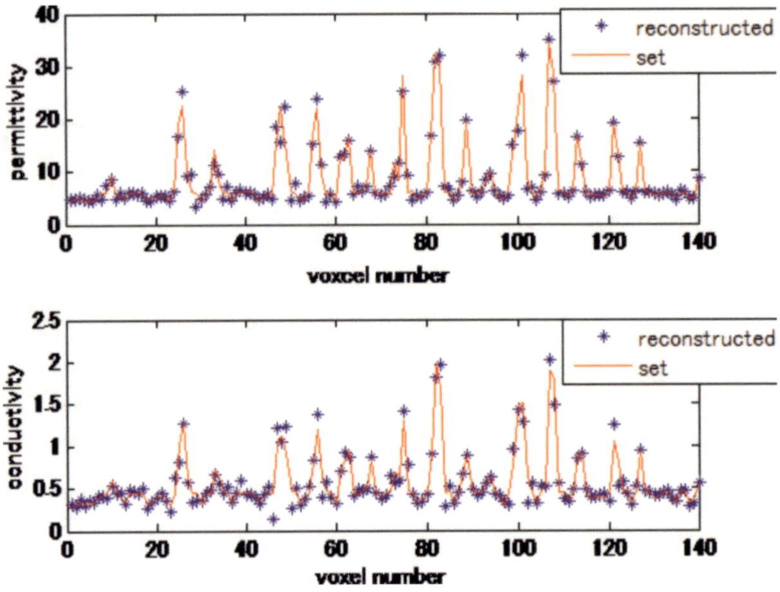

Figure 17. Quantitative evaluation of image reconstruction.

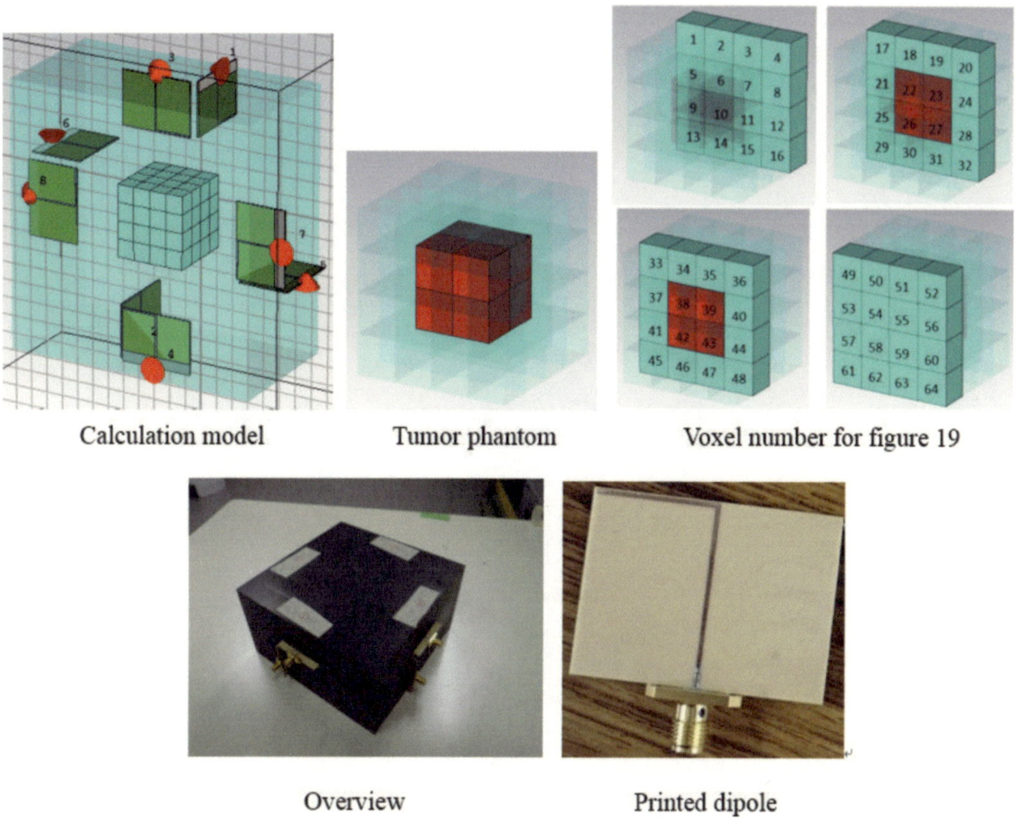

Figure 18. Experiment model.

0.75 mm are inserted into the sidewall. The polarization directions are alternated to allow robust image reconstruction. An imaging region of 40 mm × 40 mm × 40 mm is centered on the dielectric block and is discretized into 64 voxels of 10 mm × 10 mm × 10 mm. Two kinds of models are prepared. One model has an object of size 20 mm × 20 mm × 20 mm, a relative permittivity of 39.4, and conductivity of 0.9994 S/m and is placed at the center of the imaging region. This object simulates a tumor. The other model has no tumor. The measurement frequency is 1.8 GHz. In this model, 8 (monostatic response) + ${}_8C_2$ (multistatic response) = 36 data points can be obtained. Data correlation between the measured and calculated data is larger than 0.99.

The reconstructed images are shown in **Figure 19**. In order to quantitatively evaluate the reconstructed images, figures that illustrate relative permittivity versus voxel number and three-dimensional images were created. The red line and blue asterisk denote the set relative permittivity and the reconstructed value, respectively. The image is completely reconstructed for a numerical experiment with no modeling and measurement error. However, using the measurement data that includes the modeling and measurement error, the image reconstruction is unsatisfactory regardless of the high data correlation.

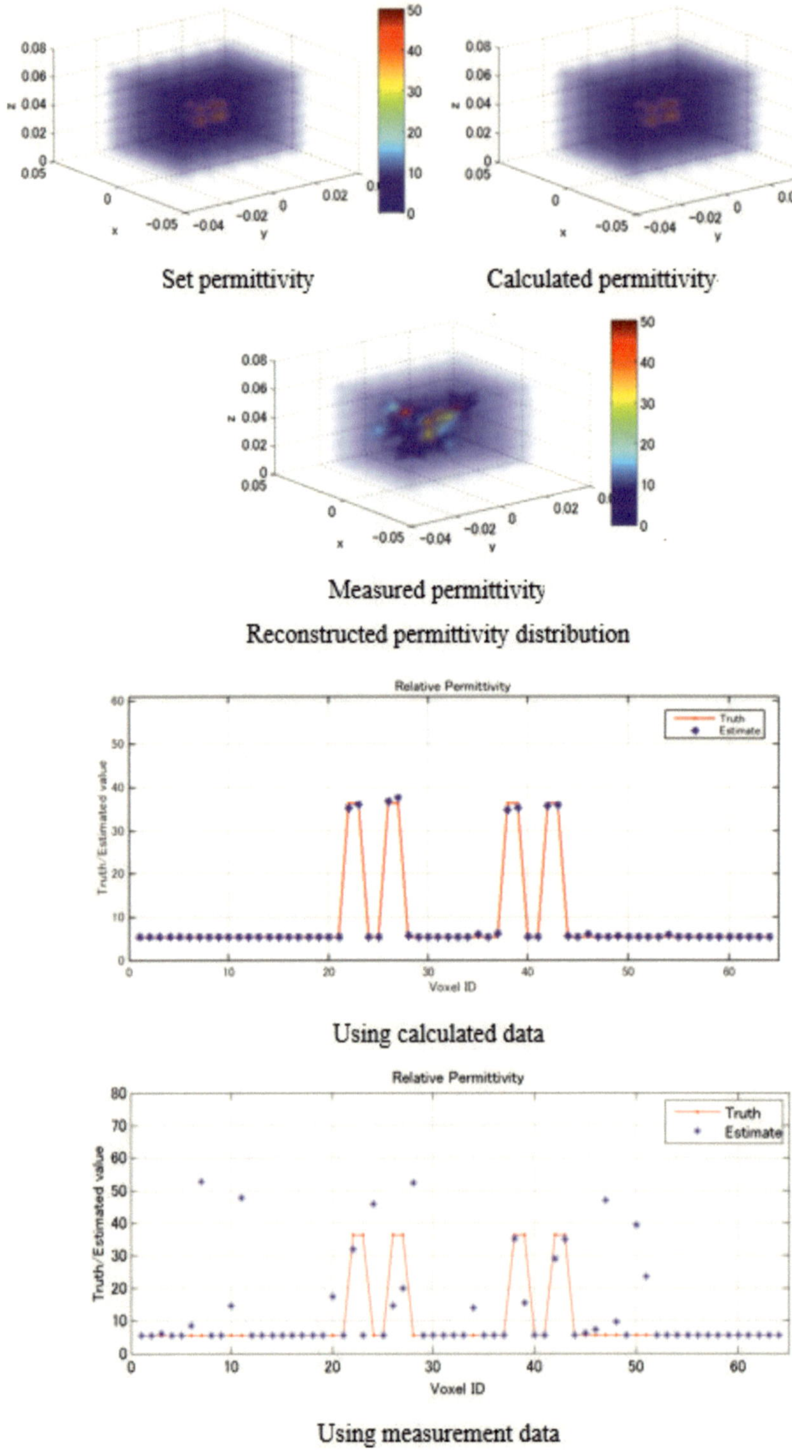

Figure 19. Image reconstruction by conventional method.

5.5. Image reconstruction by radar-assisted microwave tomography

In order to reduce the influence of errors, prior known objective shape and position assumed by the backscattered power distribution provided by the radar instead of a uniform initial distribution is introduced in the inverse scattering problem.

Figure 20 shows the backscattered power distribution using the multistatic adaptive microwave imaging (MAMI) algorithm [18]. The bandwidth is 1–3 GHz. The measured data are used for image reconstruction. The white line indicates the voxels occupied by the object. The height of each sectional view is aligned to the center level of the voxels. The backscattered power strongly corresponds to the object; thus, we can determine the outline of the object. Notably, an ordinary confocal imaging algorithm cannot provide the required image quality.

Figure 21 shows the reconstructed images using the measured data, wherein half the value of the true complex permittivity is set as the objective area. Using prior knowledge, i.e., shape and position of the object, the image can be successfully reconstructed. Although the details cannot be demonstrated owing to the limited space, the images can be reconstructed accurately under the conditions in which there is some disagreement between the scattered power distribution and the position and shape of the object.

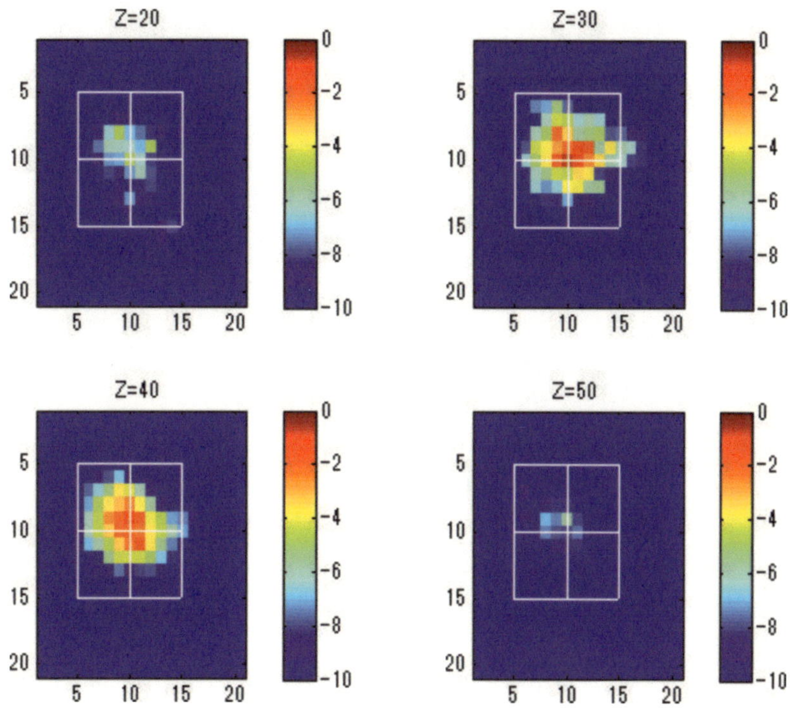

Figure 20. Backscattered power distribution by MAMI.

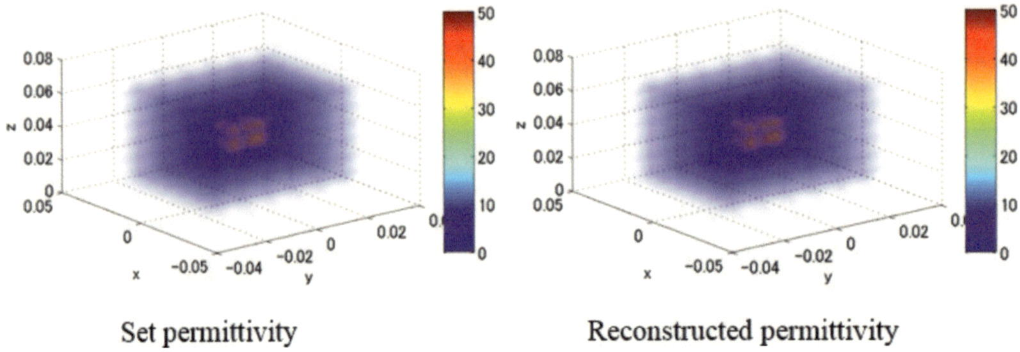

Figure 21. Image reconstruction by the proposed method.

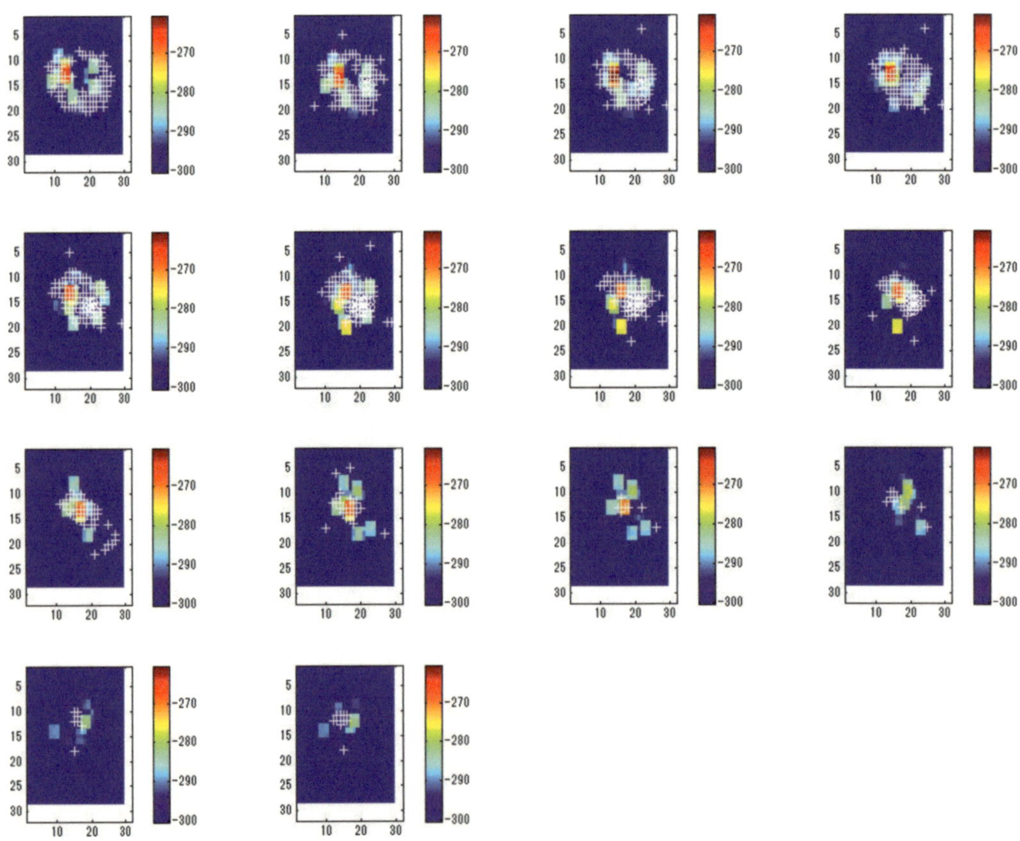

Figure 22. Numerical breast phantom imaging by MAMI.

5.6. Remarks

We have proposed a microwave tomography method using the backscattered power distribution from radar as prior knowledge. It can be confirmed through experiments that the image can be successfully reconstructed under the conditions that modeling and measurement error cannot be ignored.

One might be interested as to whether the method is effective for early breast cancer detection. **Figure 22** shows the backscattered power distribution for a complicated numerical breast phantom. The imaging sensor in **Figure 11** and MAMI were used. The bandwidth is 1–3 GHz. Symbol "+" denotes the positions of the fibroglandular tissue. A strong backscattered signal is generated around the fibroglandular tissue. Therefore, we believe that the proposed technique is effective for early breast cancer detection.

6. Conclusion: key results

Microwave tomography has the potential of a novel modality that can reconstruct both shape and property. However, it is a challenging task to develop equipment using inverse scattering program. Technologies such as sensor with breast fixing by absorption, small sensor with multipolarization, image reconstruction program linking the commercial EM simulator, hybrid imaging method using UWB radar, and inverse scattering are effective ways to aid the development.

It is also necessary to reexamine the use of radar imaging. The glandular structure in the breast is said to have strong symmetry. Using the symmetry, the presence or absence of abnormality can be detected by radar imaging. We are investigating the development of a diagnostic device that detects the presence or absence of abnormality using radar imaging and analyzes the organization properties by tomography with radar information as preliminary knowledge when the abnormality is recognized.

Author details

Yoshihiko Kuwahara

Address all correspondence to: tykuwab@ipc.shizuoka.ac.jp

Shizuoka University, Hamamatsu, Japan

References

[1] Lehman CD, Isaacs C, Schnall MD, Pisano ED, Accher SM, Weatherall DA, Bluemke DA, Bowen DJ, Marcom PK, Armstrong DK, Domchek SM, Tomlinson G, Skates SJ, Gatsonis C. Cancer yield of mammography, MR, and US in high risk women. Radiology. 2007;**224** (2):8. DOI: 10.1148/radiol.2442060461

[2] Nikolova NK. Microwave imaging for breast cancer. IEEE Microwave Magazine. 2011;**12** (7):17. DOI: 10.1109/MMM.2011.942702

[3] Lazebnik M, McCartney L, Popovic D, Watkins CB, Lindstorm MJ, Harter J, Sewell S, Magliocco A, Brooske JH, Okoniewski M, Hagness SC. A large scale study of the ultra wideband microwave dielectric properties of normal, benign, and malignant breast

tissues obtained from cancer surgeries. Physics Medical Biology. 2007;**52**(20):23. DOI: 10.1088/0031-9155/52/20/002

[4] Grzegorczyk TM, Meaney PM, Kaufman PA, diForio-Alexander RM, Paulsen KD. Fast 3D tomographic imaging for breast cancer detection. IEEE Transaction on Medical Imaging. 2012;**31**(8):9. DOI: 10.1109/TMI.2012.2197218

[5] Kuwahara Y, Miura S, Nishina Y, Mukumoto K, Ogura H, Sakahara H. Clinical setup of microwave mammography. IEICE Transactions on Communications. 2013;**96**(10):10

[6] Kuwahara Y, Ogura H, Sakahara H. Development of microwave mammography, consideration of clinical test. In: Microwave Workshop and Exhibition; November 28; Yokohama, Japan. IEICE APMC Japan National Committee; 2013. 4 p

[7] Kuwahara Y, Suzuki K, Horie H. Conformal array antenna with aspirator for microwave mammography. In: IEEE International Symposium on Antennas and Propagation, July 13, Toronto. IEEE; 2010. p. 234.11. DOI: 10.1109/APS.2010.5561879

[8] Mohamed L, Kuwahara Y. Study of correlation coefficient for breast tumor detection in microwave tomography. Open Journal Antennas and Propagation. 2015;**3**(4):10. DOI: 10.4236/ojapr.2015.34004

[9] Kuwahara Y. Microwave mammography with a small sensor and a commercial electromagnetic simulator. In: European Microwave Conference, October 6, London; 2016. 4 p. DOI: 10.1109/EuMC.2016.7824430

[10] Kuwahara Y. Application of S parameter to the inverse scattering problem. In: European Conference on Antennas and Propagation, March 21, Paris; 2017. 4 p

[11] Ono Y, Kuwahara Y. Microwave tomography assisted by radar imaging. In: European Microwave Conference; October, Nurnberg; 2017. 4 p

[12] Shea JD, Kosmas P, Hagness SC, VanVeen BD. Three dimensional microwave imaging of realistic numerical breast phantoms via a multiple frequency inverse scattering technique. Medical Physics. 2010;**37**(8):17. DOI: 10.1118/1.3443569

[13] Mays RO, Behdad N, Hagness SC. A TSVD analysis of the impact of polarization on microwave breast imaging using an enclosed array of miniaturized patch antennas. IEEE Antennas and Wireless Propagation Letters. 2015;**14**:4. DOI: 10.1109/LAWP.2014.2365755

[14] Gabriel C, Gabriel S, Corthout E. The dielectric properties of biological tissues: 1. Literature survey. Physics Medical Biology. 1996;**41**:19

[15] Sadiku MNO, editors. Numerical Techniques in Electromagnetics with MATLAB. New York: CRC Press; 2009. 710 p

[16] Bond EJ, VanVeen BD, Hagness SC. Microwave imaging via space time beamforming for early detect of breast cancer. IEEE Transactions on Antennas and Propagation. 2003;**51** (8):16. DOI: 10.1109/TAP.2003.815446

[17] Klemm M, Creddock IJ, Leenderts JA, Preece A, Gibbins DR, Share M, Benjami R. Clinical trials of a UWB imaging radar for breast cancer. In: European Conference on Antennas and Propagation, 12–16 April, Barcelona, IEEE; 2010. p. 4

[18] Xie Y, Guo B, Xu L, Li J, Stocia P. Multiple adaptive microwave imaging for early breast cancer detection. IEEE Transaction on Biomedical Engineering. 2006;**53**(8):11. DOI: 10.1109/ICASSP.2006.1660407

Chapter 4

Microwave Breast Imaging Techniques and Measurement Systems

Lulu Wang, Hu Peng and Jianhua Ma

Additional information is available at the end of the chapter

http://dx.doi.org/10.5772/intechopen.69199

Abstract

Electromagnetic waves at microwave frequencies allow penetration into many optically non-transparent mediums such as biological tissues. Over the past 30 years, researchers have extensively investigated microwave imaging (MI) approaches including imaging algorithms, measurement systems and applications in biomedical fields, such as breast tumor detection, brain stroke detection, heart imaging and bone imaging. Successful clinical trials of MI for breast imaging brought worldwide excitation, and this achievement further confirmed that the MI has potential to become a low-risk and cost-effective alternative to existing medical imaging tools such as X-ray mammography for early breast cancer detection. This chapter offers comprehensive descriptions of the most important MI approaches for early breast cancer detection, including reconstruction procedures and measurement systems as well as apparatus.

Keywords: microwave imaging, breast imaging, breast cancer detection, dielectric properties

1. Introduction

Medical imaging approaches, such as X-ray mammography, ultrasound and magnetic resonance imaging (MRI), play an important role in breast cancer detection [1]. X-ray mammography is the gold-standard method for breast cancer detection, but it has some limitations [2, 3], including harmful radiation, relatively high false-negative rates particularly with patients with dense breast tissue. Ultrasound presents good soft tissue contrast but fails in the presence of bone and air, and the image quality highly depends on operator [4]. MRI allows physicians to evaluate various parts of human body and determine the presence of certain diseases [5], but it is too expensive [6]. Therefore, it is important and necessary to develop a new imaging technique for early breast cancer detection.

In the late 1970s, Larsen et al. obtained the first microwave image of canine kidney [7]. Since then, MI has been intensively studied by many research groups [8–18], and the research objectives have been moved from imaging of organs to application-specific imaging for various tissues such as breast, joint tissues, blood and soft tissues. MI has been recommended as a safe, low-cost and low health risk alternative to existing medical imaging techniques including X-ray mammography and ultrasound. In the past many years, people paid too much attention to the MI algorithms. Several algorithms have been developed and validated numerically and in laboratory environments but they have not extensively validated in clinical environments. Recent clinical trial results demonstrated that more attention should be paid to the hardware implementation system, especially microwave sensors and sensor arrays, in clinical environments rather than laboratory environments.

This chapter presents the basic ideas of MI including currently available breast imaging methods which have been considered as important approaches for early breast cancer detection. The starting point for the development of MI methods is the formulation of the electromagnetic inverse scattering problem. Inverse scattering-based procedures address the data inversion in several different ways, depending on the target itself or on the imaging configuration and operation conditions. In this chapter, electrical properties of biological tissues, MI approaches and biomedical applications and several proof-of-concept apparatuses, including advantages, challenges and possible solutions, as well as future research directions are addressed.

2. Dielectric properties of biological tissues

The dielectric properties (DPs, relative permittivity ε_r and conductivity σ) of malignant tissues at the microwave spectrum change significantly compared to the normal tissue and the dielectric contrast can be detected and imaged by applying MI approaches [19]. The DPs of different types of biological tissues are very different due to water content difference, which are strongly nonlinear functions with frequency [20]. Choosing suitable operating frequencies for the MI system is a critical task, and the attenuation of RF signals increases with frequency due to increase in the conductivity, resulting in a lower penetration depth. Several computer models have been developed to investigate biological tissues. Debye and Cole-Cole models are the most commonly used models. The Debye model simulates the frequency dependence of DPs of tissues sufficiently [21]:

$$\varepsilon_r = \varepsilon_\infty + \frac{\varepsilon_s + \varepsilon_\infty}{1 + j\omega\tau} - j\frac{\sigma}{\omega\varepsilon_0} \quad (1)$$

where ε_∞ means the permittivity value of the tissue, ε_s is the static permittivity of the tissue, and τ is characteristic relaxation time of the medium.

Cole-Cole model is defined as [22]:

$$\varepsilon^*(\omega) = \varepsilon_\infty + \frac{\varepsilon_s - \varepsilon_\infty}{1 + (j\omega\tau)^{1-\alpha}} \quad (2)$$

where ε^* is the complex dielectric constant, ε_s and ε_∞ are static and infinite frequency dielectric constants, ω is the angular frequency and τ is a time constant. The exponent parameter α, which takes a value between 0 and 1, describes different spectral shapes. When $\alpha = 0$, the Cole-Cole model becomes to the Debye model.

Many research groups have investigated DPs of various biological tissues, including breast, heart, skin, liver, bone and lymph nodes [23–31]. Some factors that make effects on DPs of tissues include water content [20], change in the dielectric relaxation time [30], charging of the cell membrane [31], sodium content [31] and necrosis and inflammation causing breakdown of cell membrane [32].

3. Microwave imaging techniques

MI approaches can be classified as passive and active. Passive MI approaches use radiometric to measure temperature differences between normal and malignant tissues and identify the lesions based on the measurement differences. Active MI approaches span the high-MHz to low-GHz regime and appear to offer excellent opportunities to supplement the arsenal of screening tools to the radiologist, despite the fact that MI has yet to reach any demonstrated level of clinical feasibility [33]. This chapter focuses on active MI including tomography and radar-based techniques.

3.1. Microwave tomographic (MWT)

Microwave tomographic (MWT) provides quantitative information of DPs of the imaged object, which makes it possible to identify tissues and materials. One of the major limitations is heavy computation work. Based on the operating frequency of the measurement system, MMT can be grouped as single-frequency and multi-frequency approaches.

Larsen et al. [17] developed the first MWT system to produce a microwave canine kidney image at a frequency of 3.5GHz. The system consisted of one transmitting antenna and one receiving antenna, and antennas and the imaged object were immersed in coupling medium that made of water. During data collection, antennas moved to different positions. Such design was not convenient for practical implantation of MI theory, and long data acquisition time was required. To solve this problem, Hawley et al. [34] developed a new MWT system to measure blood content changes. This system consisted of a circular array of 64 waveguide antennas at an operating frequency of 2.45GHz, each waveguide antenna worked as transmitter and receiver, and mechanical movement was not required in the data collection.

A multi-frequency MWT system for breast cancer detection was developed by Meaney et al. (see **Figure 1**) [35]. The system was made of a cylindrical array of 16 monopole antennas that were placed around a breast phantom. The space between breast phantom and antennas was filled of matching medium that was made from glycerin and water mixture. This system was validated on various numerical breast models and phantoms, and simulation results showed that a small tumor (2 mm in diameter) can be imaged. A good agreement between simulation

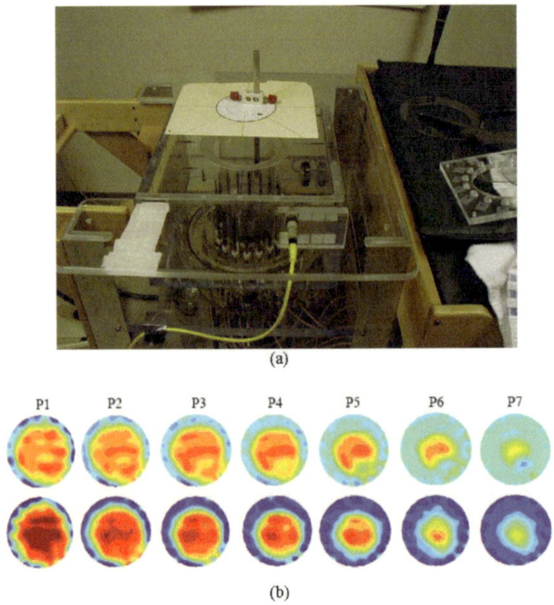

Figure 1. (a) Multi-frequency MWT system for breast cancer detection and (b) microwave (top row, permittivity, and bottom row, conductivity, at 1100 MHz) images in the same anatomically coronal view for the left breast of a woman with fatty to scattered radiographic density. P1–P7 indicates microwave tomograms spaced 1 cm apart beginning near the chest wall.

and experimental results was observed. The same research group also conducted a three-dimensional MWT system for clinical trial, and results showed that breast tumor as small as 1 cm in diameter could be detected [11]. Although clinical results did not achieve a good agreement with experimental results [35], their studies confirmed that it is possible to use MI for breast cancer detection.

3.2. Radar-based microwave imaging

Radar-based MI approaches can be classified into five groups: confocal microwave imaging (CMI), tissue sensing adaptive radar (TSAR), microwave imaging via space time (MIST), multi-static adaptive (MSA) MI, and holographic microwave imaging technique (HMI). This section presents various radar-based MI approaches for breast cancer detection.

A CMI system was developed by Hagness et al. [13, 14]. In their numerical studies, an array of 17 monopole transceivers was placed along the surface of breast model, and all antennas were equally spaced and spanning 8 cm. Results showed that a small tumor (2 mm in diameter) can be detected by using the 2D system [13], and a tumor with size of 6 mm in diameter can be detected by using the 3D system [14]. The CMI provides necessary imaging resolution and adequate penetration depth in the breast. It does not compensate for frequency-dependent propagation effects but has limited ability to discriminate against artefacts and noise. To overcome these challenges, they applied delay multiply-and-sum signal processing with CMI, where the scattered signals were time-shifted, multiplied in pair and the products were summed to form a synthetic focal point [15]. This method has an ability to produce higher resolution image and high interference rejection capability [16].

A TSAR prototype system as shown in **Figure 2(a)** was developed by Fear et al. [18]. During data acquisition, a patient was lying in prone position on the examination table with her breast extending through the breast hole and the antennas was scanned around the breast. In order to reduce the noise, the breast image was formed from the reflection signals without skin reflections. Clinical results (see **Figure 2(b)**) showed that the TSAR has an ability to detect and localize lesions with size greater than 4 mm in diameter. The major limitations of TSAR include the large reflections caused from the skin and expensive electronics for real-time imaging. To solve these problems, a Bayesian estimator was applied to enhance the reconstructed image [36].

A MIST beam-forming was developed by Bond et al. [16, 37–38]. A planar array of 16 horn antennas was placed close to the surface of the breast model, and a UWB signal was transmitted sequentially from each antenna. Numerical results demonstrated that a small tumor (2 mm in diameter) embedded in the heterogeneous breast tissue were successfully detected even with denser breast tissue. MIST offers significant improvement in performance over UWB MI approaches based on simpler focusing schemes. However, the system caused skin-breast artefacts in the image prior. The research team upgraded the imaging system (see **Figure 3(a)**) to overcome the challenges of detecting, localizing and resolving multiple or multifocal lesions [39]. The experimental results demonstrated that tumors with size of 4 mm in diameter could be imaged (see **Figure 3(b)**).

Recently, Smith et al. [40–43] proposed a near-field indirect HMI method, which involves recording the holographic intensity pattern and reconstructing the image by using Fourier transformation from the recorded intensity pattern. Compared to TSAR, indirect HMI has the ability to produce real-time image at a significantly low cost. However, more validation works are required on the theory and proof-of-concept for medical applications.

More recently, the authors proposed a far-field HMI method for imaging of biological objects [44–46]. Different from IHM, the 3D HMI uses physical displacement (scan of the distance)

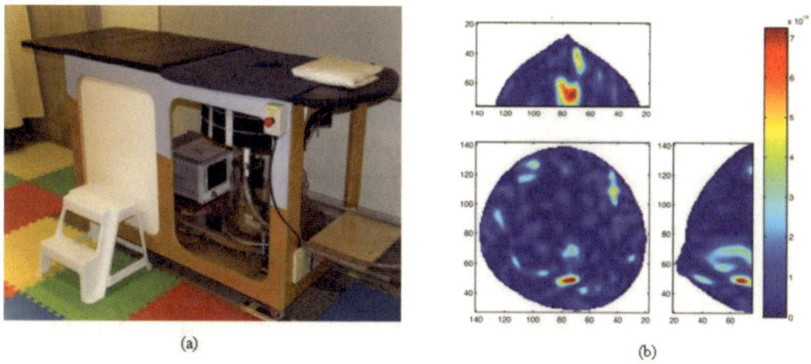

Figure 2. (a) TSAR prototype system and (b) TSAR images for patient.

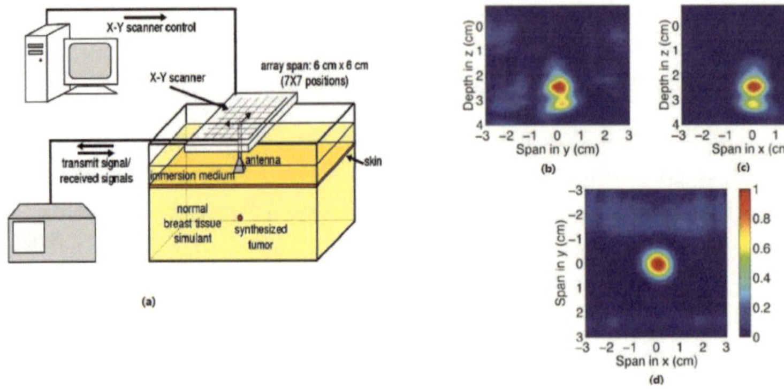

Figure 3. (a) MIST experimental system setup; reconstructed images with a 4-mm-diameter tumor; (b) yz-plane at x = 0.1 cm; (c) xz-plane at y = 0.1 cm and (d) xy-plane at z = 2.3 cm [39].

between the sensor array plane and the imaged object over a specified range (vertical) to obtain the depth information from sequenced 2D images. Both simulation and experimental results demonstrated that the HMI has several advantages in data collection, including that no matching medium was required and that the complex permittivity of the object was not required to calculate to generate an image that reduced the imaging reconstruction time.

3.3. Imaging systems

Most of existing active MI measurement systems involve hardware and software parts. The hardware system generally includes a microwave source generator, transmitting antenna(s) to send microwave signals toward the target object, receiving antennas(s) to measure the scattered electric field from the target object, a signal measurement controller to control antennas and antenna array plane, and a host computer that contains a matched software system to analyze the measured data using image processing algorithm to display the reconstructed image on a screen displaying unit. The transmitter and receiver can use the same sensor. The requirements for the hardware systems and the computational power are different due to the image algorithm differences. **Table 1** presents various developed MI systems.

3.3.1. Microwave sensor

To design an efficient and robust MI system, it is necessary to develop a sensor to match specific requirements including operating frequency, bandwidth, directivity, sensitivity, accuracy of the detection and many other factors such as compact size and low cost. Sensors should be designed specifically for lower frequencies to enhance electric field intensities inside biological tissues, due to more penetration inside the tissue when the frequency is relatively low; thus, more useful information of the object can be obtained. Various sensors have been developed for imaging of breast, including open-ended coaxial probe [47–57], tapered slot antenna (TSA) [59–63], bow-tie antenna [64–70], monopole antenna [71–78], dipole antenna [79, 80], waveguide antenna [81–84], patch antenna and Vivaldi antenna.

	Dartmouth College (USA)	Keele University (UK)	University of Bristol (UK)	University of Manitoba (Canada)	Auckland University of Technology (NZ)
Antenna	Circular array of 16 monopoles	Circular array of 24 ceramic-filled open-ended waveguides	Two spherical arrays consist of 31 and 60 ultra-wideband antennas	Circular array of doubled layers Vivaldi antennas	Spiral array of 16 open-ended waveguide antennas
Frequency	0.5–3 GHz	1.0–2.3 GHz	4–8 GHz	3–6 GHz	12 GHz
Test phantom	Real patients	Soft animal tissues	Real breasts	Various dielectric objects	Various dielectric objects
Immersion medium	0.9% saline ($\varepsilon_r = 76.6$, $\Sigma = 2.48$ S/m)	Metallic bath with coupling liquid	Matching ceramic	No matching medium, air only	No matching medium, air
Image	2D and 3D	2D	3D	2D	2D and 3D
Clinical trial	Yes	No	Yes	No	No

Table 1. Various MI measurement systems.

Open-ended coaxial probes were employed in MI systems to measure dielectric properties of biological tissues [47–56]. Advantages of using probes include that tissue manipulation or preparation is not required, dielectric-properties measurements can be integrated in a straightforward manner with surgical and pathology protocols, they are easy to use, they can respond at broadband frequencies and there is a capacity for noninvasive measurements. However, accuracy and reliability of the measurements depend on the aperture of probe as it is the only part of the system in direct contact with the imaged object.

A compact tapered slot antenna (TSA) was applied in an UWB MI system by Bialkowski et al. [58], and the benefits include high directivity, wide bandwidth, simple feed structure and relatively low in cost, which makes TSA become a popular choice for implementation of MI systems [59–63].

UWB bow-tie sensors were used by John et al. [70]. The system is made of an imaging cavity formed from 12 panels soldered together, and each panel is made of three UWB bow-tie sensors as shown in **Figure 4**. The coupling medium was filled in the cavity, and an image of a spherical object was reconstructed by using inverse scattering algorithm. Advantages of using bow-tie sensor include compact, wideband and easy-to-manufacture.

Researchers at Dartmouth College developed an MWT system that is made of a cylindrical array of 16 monopole antennas (see **Figure 1**), one antenna acting as transmitter and others acting as receivers, and sensors were placed in a coupling medium that is made of material close to fatty tissues. The system was validated on breast phantoms and real human subjects [35]. Advantages of using monopole antennas include easy to model, compact, can be placed at different geometries and can be impedance-matched across a wide bandwidth when immersed in a lossy medium.

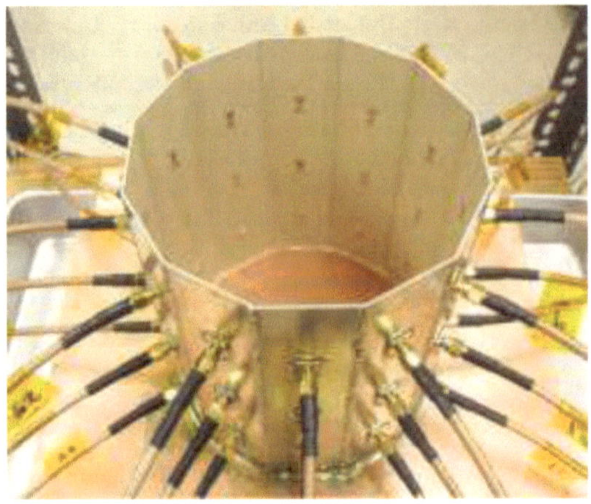

Figure 4. Imaging cavity demonstrated in John's publication [82].

Open-ended waveguide antennas were applied in the HMI system by the authors [46]. The HMI system was made of an array of 16 open-ended waveguide antennas, one acting as transmitter and other being receivers. During data collection, the transmitter continuously generated RF signals to the breast phantom and the scattered electric fields were measured by receivers. No matching medium was required in this measurement system.

3.3.2. *Microwave sensor array*

Investigators also studied the performance of producing high-resolution images at lower costs, including image algorithms, sensor design and sensor array geometry. People paid much attention to image algorithm and sensor design, but very little attentions have been paid to sensor arrays and their applications in the biomedical field. Most of the existing MI systems use circular- [18], planar- [38] and spherical [85]-shaped sensor array. The circular sensor array is more suitable for clinical settings. To generate a high-resolution image, a large number of sensors (from several to several hundreds) are required for the existing MI system. The image is improved with increasing the total number of sensors used in the system. However, limitations of increasing sensor numbers include the increased cost, size and complexity.

Recently, Klemm et al. [85] proposed a spherical array of 16 patch antennas for the clinical applicable CMI system. During data collection, the patient was lying in a prone position, which was felt to offer the best chance of the breast forming a gentle and uniformly curved shape. Experimental results showed that the image quality can be improved by improving the bandwidth of the array element.

More recently, the authors [46] proposed a spiral and random sensor array that contains 16 waveguide antennas for HMI system as shown in **Figure 5**. The experimental results showed that the breast phantom image can be improved by using spiral and random sensor arrays compared to the regular spaced sensor array. Color bar plots signal intensity on a linear scale.

http://dx.doi.org/10.5772/intechopen.69199

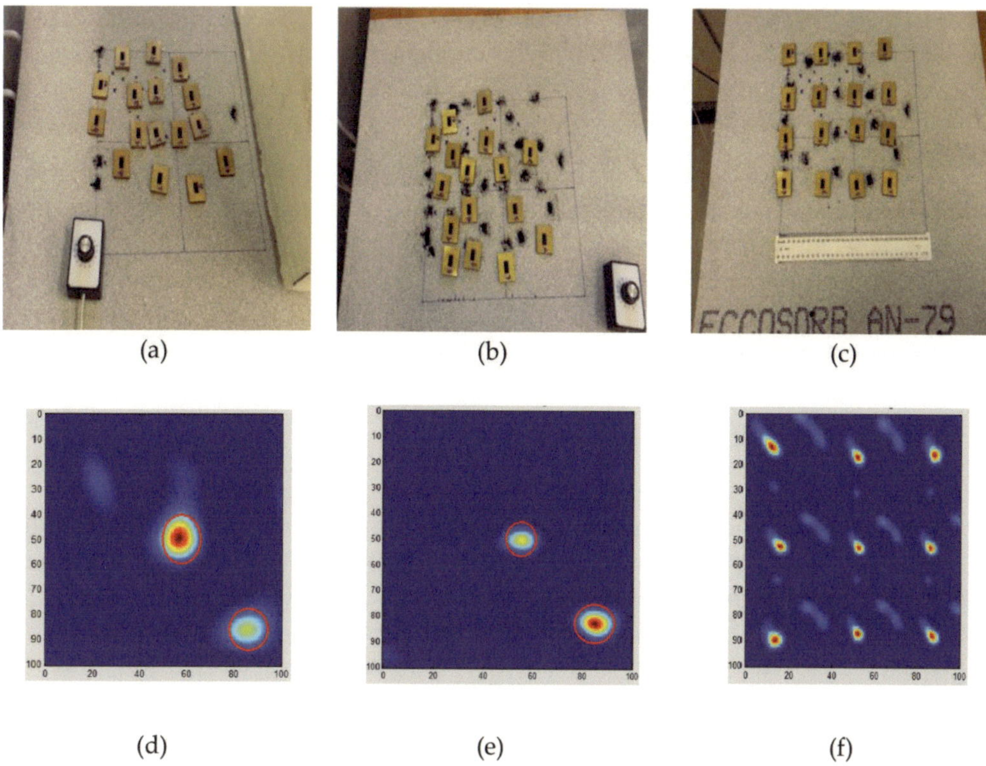

Figure 5. (a) Spiral array; (b) random array; (c) regularly spaced; reconstructed images of two inclusions using (d) spiral array; (e) random array and (f) regularly spaced array.

4. Challenges and future work

There are several major limitations for practical implementations of MI approaches. First, breast phantoms were made of simple materials, which cannot represent real human tissues accurately. Second, the electrical properties contrasts between the normal and the malignant tissues are much smaller than people thought, which caused more difficultly in imaging the structures. Choosing a suitable operating frequency range is also a challenging task. These challenges can be solved by developing a high dynamic system to capture the small difference in the scattered field or by developing a contrast agent to enhance the electrical properties of the malignant tissues. The spatial resolution is another major challenge. To enhance spatial resolution of an MI system, many researchers increased the number of microwave sensors for the implementation system. For example, the sensor number has been increased from 16 to 256 to increase the image quality [86]. However, the detection accuracy may be reduced due to the mutual coupling signals produced between sensors. Moreover, the system became very complex and the implementation costs increased significantly.

To address these problems, one single scanning antenna may be used instead of several antennas. Investigation of sensor arrays such as unequally spaced sensor arrays and applying compressive sensing approach [87, 88] may be another solution. Some recently proposed techniques such as multiple-input-multiple-output technique [89] may be able to reduce the complexity of the system. Finally, most of the existing experimental systems require the coupling medium between sensors and the imaged object, which increased the system cost significantly.

Many promising indicators suggested that MI systems in the future will be a successful clinical complement to conventional mammography. Investigations may improve the imaging algorithms and hardware implementation systems with particular focus on highly sensitive, compact and low-cost microwave sensors and sensor arrays to achieve high-quality images at relatively low cost. Significant contributions from existing MI commercial companies may be greatly helpful in developing the well-established MI modalities to clinical trials.

5. Conclusion

In conclusion, this chapter presented an exhaustive summary of MI approaches with particular focus on implementations of microwave breast imaging theory, including image algorithms, experimental setups, microwave sensors and sensor arrays. Several MI implementation apparatuses were reviewed in detail. MI systems have direct impacts on spatial resolution, operating frequencies, detection accuracy and quality of imaging. Several advantages of existing MI approaches, open challenges, possible solutions and future research directions were also discussed. Successful clinical trials of MI for breast imaging made the worldwide excitation, and this achievement confirmed that MI has potential to become a low-risk alternative to existing medical imaging tools such as X-ray mammography for breast cancer detection. However, MI-based techniques are still far from maturity due to the fact that many challenges have to be addressed before MI can be implemented in clinical environments.

Acknowledgements

This work was supported in part by the National Natural Science Foundation of China (NSFC) under Grant 61701159, in part by the Natural Science Foundation of Anhui Province under Grant 101413246, in part by the Foundation for Oversea Master Project from the Ministry of Education, China, under Grant 2160311028, and in part by the start-up funding from the Hefei University of Technology under Grant 407037164.

Author details

Lulu Wang[1]*, Hu Peng[1] and Jianhua Ma[2]

*Address all correspondence to: luluwang2015@hfut.edu.cn

1 School of Instrument Science and Opto-electronics Engineering, Hefei University of Technology, Hefei, China

2 School of Biomedical Technology, Southern Medical University, Guangzhou, China

References

[1] Fass L. Imaging and cancer: A review. Molecular Oncology. 2008;**2**(2):115-152

[2] Kerlikowske K, Gard CC, Sprague BL, Tice JA, Miglioretti DL. One vs. two breast density measures to predict 5- and 10-year breast cancer risk. Cancer Epidemiology, Biomarkers and Prevention: A Publication of the American Association for Cancer Research, Cosponsored by the American Society of Preventive Oncology. 2005; **24**(6):889

[3] O'Halloran M, Conceicao RC, Byrne D, Glavin M, Jones E. FDTD modeling of the breast: A review. Progress in Electromagnetics Research B. 2009;**18**:1-24

[4] Chan V, Perlas A. Basics of Ultrasound Imaging. New York: Springer; 2011

[5] Jacobs MA, Ibrahim TS, Ouwerkerk R. MR imaging: Brief overview and emerging applications. Radiographics. 2007;**274**:1213-1229

[6] Baltzer PA, Benndorf M, Dietzel M, Gajda M, Runnebaum IB, Kaiser WA. False-positive findings at contrast-enhanced breast mri: A bi-rads descriptor study. Breast Diseases: A Year Book Quarterly. 2011;**22**(1):44-45

[7] Wang Z, Lim EG, Tang Y, Leach M. Medical applications of microwave imaging. IEEE Press, New York, 1985.

[8] Fallahpour M, Case JT, Ghasr M, Zoughi R. Piecewise and Wiener filter-based SAR techniques for monostatic microwave imaging of layered structures. IEEE Transactions on Antennas and Propagation. 2014;**62**(1):1-13

[9] De Zaeytijd J, Franchois A, Eyraud C, Geffrin JM. Fullwave three-dimensional microwave imaging with a regularized Gauss–Newton method—Theory and experiment. IEEE Transactions on Antennas and Propagation. 2007;**55**(11):3279-3292

[10] Chandra R, Zhou H, Balasingham I, Narayanan RM. On the opportunities and challenges in microwave medical sensing and imaging. IEEE Transactions on Biomedical Engineering. 2015;**62**(7):1667-1682

[11] Meaney PM, Goodwin D, Golnabi A, Zhou T, Pallone M, Geimer S, Burke G, Paulsen K. Clinical microwave tomographic imaging of the calcaneus: A first-in-human case study of two subjects. IEEE Transactions on Biomedical Engineering. 2012;**59**(12): 3304-3313

[12] Semenov SY, Corfield DR. Microwave tomography for brain imaging: Feasibility assessment for stroke detection. International Journal of Antennas and Propagation. 2008;2548301-2548308

[13] Shea JD, Hagness SC, Van Veen BD. Hardware acceleration of FDTD computations for 3-D microwave breast tomography. IEEE Antennas and Propagation Society International Symposium. 2009. pp. 1-4

[14] Mashal A, Sitharaman B, Li X, Avti PK. Toward carbon-nanotube-based theranostic agents for microwave detection and treatment of breast cancer: Enhanced dielectric and heating response of tissue-mimicking materials. IEEE Transactions on Biomedical Engineering. 2010;**57**(8):1831

[15] Van Veen BD, Hagness SC, Bond EJ, Li X. Space-time microwave imaging for cancer detection. US Patent. 2009;US 7570063 B2

[16] Koutsoupidou M, Karanasiou IS, Kakoyiannis CG, Groumpas E, Conessa C, Joachimowicz N. Evaluation of a tumor detection microwave system with a realistic breast phantom. Microwave and Optical Technology Letters. 2017;**59**(1):6-10

[17] Mohammed AM, Abbosh S, Mustafa D, Ireland D. Microwave system for head imaging. IEEE Transactions on Instrumentation and Measurement. 2014;**63**(1):117-123

[18] Fear EC, Bourqui J, Curtis C, Mew D. Microwave breast imaging with a monostatic radar-based system: A study of application to patients. IEEE Transactions on Microwave Theory and Techniques. 2013;**61**(5):2119-2128

[19] Schulz S, Pusch S, Pohl E, Dielkus S, Herbst-Irmer R, Meller A. Investigation of tumor using an antenna scanning system. IEEE Microwave Symposium. 2014;**171**:1401-1406

[20] Lazebnik M, Watkins CB, Hagness SC, Booske JH. The dielectric properties of normal and malignant breast tissue at microwave frequencies: Analysis, conclusions, and implications from the Wisconsin/Calgary study. IEEE Antennas and Propagation Society International Symposium. 2007. pp. 2172-2175

[21] Lazebnik M, Okoniewski M, Booske JH, Hagness SC. Highly accurate Debye models for normal and malignant breast tissue dielectric properties at microwave frequencies. IEEE Microwave and Wireless Components Letters. 2007;**17**(12):822-824

[22] Said T, Varadan VV. Variation of Cole-Cole model parameters with the complex permittivity of biological tissues. In: 2009. MTT'09. IEEE MTT-S International Microwave Symposium Digest; IEEE; 2009. pp. 1445-1448

[23] Kim T, Oh J, Kim B, Lee J, Jeon S, Pack J. A study of dielectric properties of fatty, malignant and fibro-glandular tissues in female human breast. Asia-Pacific Symposium on Electromagnetic Compatibility and International Zurich Symposium on Electromagnetic Compatibility. 2008;216-219

[24] Garrett JD, Fear EC. Average dielectric property analysis of complex breast tissue with microwave transmission measurements. Sensors. 2015;**15**(15):1199-1216

[25] Fu F, Xin SX, Chen W. Temperature- and frequency-dependent dielectric properties of biological tissues within the temperature and frequency ranges typically used for magnetic resonance imaging-guided focused ultrasound surgery. International Journal of Hyperthermia. 2014;**30**(1):56

[26] O'Rourke AP, Lazebnik M, Bertram JM, Converse MC, Hagness SC, Webster JC. Dielectric properties of human normal, malignant and cirrhotic liver tissue: In vivo and

ex vivo measurements from 0.5 to 20 Ghz using a precision open-ended coaxial probe. Physics in Medicine and Biology. 2007;**52**(15):4707-4719

[27] Zhang L, Liu P, Shi X, You F, Dong X. A comparative study of a calibration method for measuring the dielectric properties of biological tissues on electrically small open-ended coaxial probe. IEEE International Conference on Biomedical Engineering and Biotechnology. 2012. pp. 658-661

[28] Zhang L, Shi X, You F, Liu P, Dong X. Improved circuit model of open-ended coaxial probe for measurement of the biological tissue dielectric properties between megahertz and gigahertz. Physiological Measurement. 2013;**34**(10):N83

[29] Yamamoto T, Koshiji K, Fukuda A. Development of test fixture for measurement of dielectric properties and its verification using animal tissues. Physiological Measurement. 2013;**34**(9):1179

[30] Lazebnik M, Mccartney L, Popovic D, Watkins CB, Lindstrom MJ, Harter J. A large-scale study of the ultrawideband microwave dielectric properties of normal, benign and malignant breast tissues obtained from cancer surgeries. Physics in Medicine and Biology. 2007;**52**(20):6093-6115

[31] Abeyrathne CD, Halgamuge MN, Farrell PM, Skafidas E. An ab-initio computational method to determine dielectric properties of biological materials. Scientific Reports. 2013;**3**(5):1796

[32] Rossmanna C, Haemmerich D. Review of temperature dependence of thermal properties, dielectric properties, and perfusion of biological tissues at hyperthermic and ablation temperatures. Critical Reviews in Biomedical Engineering. 2014;**42**(6):467-469

[33] Ibrahim WMA, Algabroun HM. The Family Tree of Breast Microwave Imaging Techniques. In: 4th Kuala Lumpur International Conference on Biomedical Engineering; Springer: Berlin Heidelberg; 2008

[34] Nikawa Y. Microwave diagnosis using MRI and image of capillary blood vessel. IEEE Asia Pacific Microwave Conference. 2009. pp. 595-598

[35] Meaney PM, Fanning MW, Raynolds T, Fox CJ, Fang Q, Kogel CA. Initial clinical experience with microwave breast imaging in women with normal mammography. Academic Radiology. 2007;**14**(2):207-218

[36] O'Halloran M, Byrne D, Elahi MA, Conceição RC, Jones E, Glavin M. Confocal Microwave Imaging. An Introduction to Microwave Imaging for Breast Cancer Detection, Part of the series Biological and Medical Physics, Biomedical Engineering. Springer International Publishing,AG Switzerland. 2016. pp. 47-73.

[37] Salvador SM, Fear EC, Okoniewski M, Matyas JR. Exploring joint tissues with microwave imaging. IEEE Transactions on Microwave Theory and Techniques. 2010;**58**(8):2307-2313

[38] Ricci E, Maggio F, Rossi T, Cianca E, Ruggieri M. UWB radar imaging based on space-time beamforming for stroke detection. IFMBE Proceedings. 2015;**45**:946-949

[39] Li X, Davis S K, Hagness S C, Van D W, Van Veen B D. Microwave imaging via space-time beam forming: Experimental investigation of tumor detection in multilayer breast phantoms. IEEE Transactions on Microwave Theory & Techniques, 2004, **52**(8):1856-1865.

[40] Smith D, Livingstone B, Elsdon M, Zheng H. The development of indirect microwave holography for measurement and imaging applications. 2015 IEEE Microwave Symposium. 2015;**722**:1-4

[41] Smith D, Yurduseven O, Livingstone B. The use of indirect holographic techniques for microwave imaging. IEEE Microwave Techniques. 2013;**10**:16-21

[42] Yurduseven O, Smith D, Livingstone B, Schejbal V, You Z. Investigations of resolution limits for indirect microwave holographic imaging. International Journal of RF and Microwave Computer-Aided Engineering. 2013;**23**(4):410-416

[43] Smith D, Yurduseven O, Livingstone B, Schejbal V. Microwave imaging using indirect holographic techniques. IEEE Antennas and Propagation Magazine. 2014;**56**(1):104-117

[44] Wang L, Al-Jumaily AM, Simpkin R. Imaging of 3-D dielectric objects using far-field holographic microwave imaging technique. Progress in Electromagnetics Research B. 2014;**61**:135-147

[45] Wang L, Al-Jumaily AM, Simpkin R. Three-dimensional far-field holographic microwave imaging: An experimental investigation of dielectric object. Progress in Electromagnetics Research B. 2014;**61**(1):169-184

[46] Wang L, Al-Jumaily AM, Simpkin R. Investigation of antenna array configurations using far-field holographic microwave imaging technique. Progress in Electromagnetics Research M. 2015;**42**:1-11

[47] Bobowski JS, Johnson T. Permittivity measurements of biological samples by an open-ended coaxial line. Progress in Electromagnetics Research B. 2012;**40**(40):159-183

[48] Reinecke T, Hagemeier L, Ahrens S, Klintschar M. Permittivity measurements for the quantification of edema in human brain tissue Open-ended coaxial and coplanar probes for fast tissue scanning. IEEE Sensors conference. 2014, Nov, 681-683

[49] Sato Y, Hirata A, Fujiwara O. In-vivo measurement of complex relative permittivity for human skin tissues using open-ended coaxial probe. IEEE Transactions on Electronics Information and Systems. 2011;**131**(131):2040-2045

[50] Huang R, Zhang D. Analysis of open-ended coaxial probes by using a two-dimensional finite-difference frequency-domain method. IEEE Transactions on Instrumentation and Measurement. 2008;**57**(5):931-939

[51] Michiyama T, Nikawa Y, Kuwano S. Measurement of complex permittivity for soft material using easy sticking open ended coaxial probe. Transactions of the Institute of Electronics Information and Communication Engineers C. 2010;**93**:167-174

[52] Jung JH, Cho JH, Kim SY. Accuracy enhancement of wideband complex permittivity measured by an open-ended coaxial probe. Measurement Science and Technology. 2016;**27**(1):015011

[53] Habibi M, Klemer DP, Raicu V. Two dimensional dielectric spectroscopy: Implementation and validation of a scanning open-ended coaxial probe. Review of Scientific Instruments. 2010;**81**(7):255-258

[54] Brusson M, Rossignol J, Binczak S, Laurent G. Determination of burn depth in the ablation of atrial fibrillation using an open-ended coaxial probe. Sensors & Actuators B Chemical. 2015, **209**: 1097-1101.

[55] Misra DK, Mckelvey JA. A quasistatic method for the characterization of stratified dielectric materials using an open-ended coaxial probe. Microwave & Optical Technology Letters. 2010;**7**(7):650-653

[56] Misra DK. Evaluation of the complex permittivity of layered dielectric materials with the use of an open-ended coaxial line. Microwave and Optical Technology Letters. 2015;**11**(11):183-187

[57] Meaney P M, Gregory A P, Epstein N R, Paulsen K D. Microwave open-ended coaxial dielectric probe: interpretation of the sensing volume re-visited. BMC Medical Physics. 2014, **14**(1):1-11.

[58] Tiang SS, Ain MF, Abdullah MZ. Compact and wideband wide-slot antenna for microwave imaging system. IEEE RF and Microwave Conference. 2011. pp. 63-66

[59] Gopikrishna M, Krishna DD, Aanandan CK, Mohanan P. Compact linear tapered slot antenna for UWB applications. Electronics Letters. 2008;**44**(20):1174-1175

[60] Costa JR, Medeiros CR, Fernandes CA. Performance of a crossed exponentially tapered slot antenna for UWB systems. IEEE Transactions on Antennas and Propagation. 2009;**57**(5):1345-1352

[61] Azim R, Islam MT, Misran N. Compact tapered-shape slot antenna for UWB applications. IEEE Antennas and Wireless Propagation Letters. 2011;**10**(3):1190-1193

[62] Wu J, Zhao Z, Liu J, Nie ZP, Liu QH. A compact linear tapered slot antenna with integrated Balun for UWB applications. Progress in Electromagnetics Research C. 2012;**29**:163-176

[63] Lu WJ, Zhang ZY, Liu R, Zhu HB. Design concept of a narrow-wideband antenna for spectrum sensing applications. IEEE China-Japan Joint Microwave Conference. 2011. pp. 1-4

[64] Mehdipour A, Mohammadpour-Aghdam K, Faraji-Dana R, Sebak AR. Modified slot bow-tie antenna for UWB applications. Microwave and Optical Technology Letters. 2008;**50**(2):429-432

[65] Hirata A. Double-sided printed bow-tie antenna with notch filter for UWB applications. Journal of Electromagnetic Waves and Applications. 2012;**23**(2):247-253

[66] Sayidmarie KH, Fadhel YA. A planar self-complementary bow-tie antenna for UWB applications. Progress in Electromagnetics Research C. 2013;**35**:253-267

[67] Kumar R, Surushe G. Design of microstrip-fed printed uwb diversity antenna with tee crossed shaped structure. Engineering Science and Technology, an International Journal. 2016;**19**(2):946-955

[68] Jalilvand M, Li X, Kowalewski J, Zwick T. Broadband miniaturised bow-tie antenna for 3D microwave tomography. Electronics Letters. 2014; **50**(4):244-246

[69] Ünal Ø, Türetken B, Canbay C, Ünal Ø, Türetken B. Spherical conformal bow-tie antenna for ultra-wide band microwave imaging of breast cancer tumor. Applied Computational Electromagnetics Society Journal. 2014;**29**(2):124-133

[70] John S, Mark H, Paul C, Mahta M. A preclinical system prototype for focused microwave thermal therapy of the breast. IEEE Transactions on Biomedical Engineering. 2012;**59**(9):2431-2438

[71] Ojaroudi M, Kohneshahri G, Noory J. Small modified monopole antenna for UWB application. IET Microwaves Antennas and Propagation. 2009;**3**(5):863-869

[72] Ni W, Nakajima N. Small printed inverted-l monopole antenna for worldwide interoperability for microwave access wideband operation. IET Microwaves Antennas and Propagation. 2010;**4**(1):1714-1719

[73] Halili K, Ojaroudi M, Ojaroudi N. Ultrawideband monopole antenna for use in a circular cylindrical microwave imaging system. Microwave and Optical Technology Letters. 2012;**54**(9):2202-2205

[74] Golezani JJ, Abbak M, Akduman I. Modified directional wide band printed monopole antenna for use in radar and microwave imaging applications. Progress in Electromagnetics Research Letters. 2012;**33**:119-129

[75] Latif S, Flores-Tapia D, Pistorius S, Shafai L. A planar ultrawideband elliptical monopole antenna with reflector for breast microwave imaging. Microwave and Optical Technology Letters. 2014;**56**(4):808-813

[76] Ojaroudi N, Ojaroudi M, Ebazadeh Y. UWB/omni-directional microstrip monopole antenna for microwave imaging applications. Progress in Electromagnetics Research C. 2014;**47**:139-146

[77] Ojaroudi N, Ojaroudi M, Ghadimi N. UWB omnidirectional square monopole antenna for use in circular cylindrical microwave imaging systems. Wireless Personal Communications. 2015;**11**(3):1350-1353

[78] Ojaroudi M, Civi OA. Bandwidth enhancement of small square monopole antenna using self-complementary structure for microwave imaging system applications. Applied Computational Electromagnetics Society Journal. 2015;**30**(12):1360-1365

[79] Saenz E, Guven K, Ozbay E, Ederra I, Gonzalo P. Decoupling of multifrequency dipole antenna arrays for microwave imaging applications. International Journal of Antennas and Propagation. 2010;**4**:252-260

[80] Ahdi Rezaeieh S, Bialkowski K, Zamani A, Abbosh A. Loop-dipole composite antenna for wideband microwave-based medical diagnostic systems with verification on pulmonary edema detection. IEEE Antennas and Wireless Propagation Letters. 2015;**15**:1

[81] Ali M, Tailor A. Broadband coplanar waveguide-fed slot antenna for wireless local area networks and microwave imaging applications. Microwave and Optical Technology Letters. 2007;**49**(4):846-852

[82] Saleh W, Qaddoumi N. Potential of near-field microwave imaging in breast cancer detection utilizing tapered rectangular waveguide probes. Computers and Electrical Engineering. 2009;**35**(4):587-593

[83] Diener L. Microwave near-field imaging with open-ended waveguide—Comparison with other techniques of nondestructive testing. Research in Nondestructive Evaluation. 2009;**7**(2-3):137-152

[84] Brovko AV, Murphy EK, Yakovlev VV. Waveguide microwave imaging: Neural network reconstruction of functional 2-D permittivity profiles. IEEE Transactions on Microwave Theory and Techniques. 2009;**57**(2):406-414

[85] Klemm M, Craddock IJ, Leendertz JA, Preece A. Radar-Based breast cancer detection using a hemispherical antenna array-experimental results. IEEE Transactions on Antennas and Propagation. 2009;**57**(6):1692-1704

[86] Kurrant D, Bourqui J, Curtis C, Fear E. Evaluation of 3d acquisition surfaces for radar-based microwave breast imaging. IEEE Transactions on Antennas and Propagation. 2015;**63**(11):1-1

[87] Craven D, O'Halloran M, Mcginley B, Conceicao RC, Kilmartin L, Jones E. Compressive sampling for time critical microwave imaging applications. Healthcare Technology Letters. 2014;**1**(1):6-12

[88] Bevacqua MT, Scapaticci R. A compressive sensing approach for 3D breast cancer microwave imaging with magnetic nanoparticles as contrast agent. IEEE Transactions on Medical Imaging. 2016;**35**(2):665-673

[89] Qi Y. Application of sparse array and MIMO in near-range microwave imaging. Proceedings of SPIE - The International Society for Optical Engineering. 2011;**8179**(4): 81790X-81790X-12

Chapter 5

Advances in Breast Thermography

Siva Teja Kakileti, Geetha Manjunath,
Himanshu Madhu and
Hadonahalli Venkataramanappa Ramprakash

Additional information is available at the end of the chapter

http://dx.doi.org/10.5772/intechopen.69198

Abstract

Thermography-based breast cancer screening has several advantages as it is non-contact, non-invasive and safe. Many clinical trials have shown its effectiveness to detect cancer earlier than any other modality. Historically, thermography has only been used as an adjunct modality due to the high expertise required for manual interpretation of the thermal images and high false-positive rates otherwise found in general use. Recent developments in thermal sensors, image capture protocols and computer-aided software diagnostics are showing great promise in making this modality a mainstream cancer screening method. This chapter describes some of these advances in breast thermography and computer-aided diagnostics that are poised to improve the quality of cancer care.

Keywords: breast cancer, thermography, analytics, machine learning, artificial intelligence, medical imaging, breast thermography, computer-aided diagnostics

1. Introduction

Breast cancer is the leading cause of cancer deaths in women today. According to WHO, 1 in every 12 women have the risk of a breast abnormality in her lifetime. It is well established that early diagnosis is very critical to increase survival rates. For example, a study sponsored by Australian Government found that the breast cancer survival is strongly associated with tumor size at detection. In Australia in 1997, five-year relative survival was 98, 95, 93, 88 and 73% for women with tumors of size 0–10, 11–15, 16–19, 20–29 and 30 mm or greater, respectively [1]. Unfortunately, 70% of the breast cancer cases are detected when the tumor size is over 30 mm [2]. Therefore, there is a critical need for a method that can detect early-stage breast cancer.

Thermography is a method of cancer screening that has been known to detect early-stage cancer [3]. However, there is a lot of variation in the results of clinical studies based on thermography and many show low specificity. A medical scientist and deep expert in thermography, Dr. Gautherie, observed that the lack of technical skill and expertise to interpret thermal images leads to this low diagnostic accuracy [3]. Recent developments on high-resolution thermal cameras and computer algorithms for thermal analysis are making the interpretation process more factual. With increased computation power, automated diagnostics is also able to decrease the false-positive rates. Hence, thermal imaging along with computer-aided diagnostics is showing a promise of upgrading breast thermography to main stream usage. In this chapter, we study these recent trends in advanced thermal imaging as well as the advances in imaging algorithms.

2. Introduction to thermography

Infrared thermography is the recording of temperature distribution of a body using the infrared radiation emitted by the surface of that body at wavelengths between 7 and 14 μm. With this information, it is possible to create a visual map or thermogram of the distribution of temperatures on the surface of the object imaged. The sensitivity of modern infrared cameras is such that temperature differences to 0.025°C can be detected.

Thermography can be used for breast cancer screening based on the fact that the temperature of the tumor is about 2°C higher than the neighboring tissues and blood vessel activity surrounding a developing cancer is almost always higher than in normal breast tissue. Since breast tissue is part of the skin, vascular alterations due to cancer result in temperature changes on the surface of the breast which can be captured with infrared thermography. Thermal abnormalities identified with thermal imaging are among the earliest signs of a pre-cancerous or cancerous lesion of the breast.

Thermal imaging is a noncontact, noninvasive and extremely privacy aware. Since thermal cameras are small, they are very portable and can be used for screening in rural camps.

There are many certified thermographers and thermologists who continue to practice using thermal analysis for breast cancer diagnosis [4].

3. Comparison with mammography

Most common methods used for cancer screening today is clinical examination, mammography and ultrasound. Among them, mammography is considered as a gold standard for breast cancer screening. It uses X-rays to screen the breast region and digitizes the density difference in image format. Typically, cancerous tumor has high density compared to surrounding region and can be easily distinguished from other regions. Studies [5–7] show that it gives a sensitivity of 68% to 88% (or as low as 48% for extremely dense breasts) and specificities ranging from 82% to 98%. In addition, it has the following disadvantages:

1. *Low sensitivity toward younger women:* In order to clearly detect tumors using X-rays, the density of the lump should be higher than the surrounding tissue density. Breast tissue density in younger women is high and decreases with age and exposure to hormonal changes [8]. This makes mammography mainly applicable for women with age greater than 45 years.
2. *Risk of radiation:* X-rays can cause genetic change in the tissues, and these mutations increase with increased dosage of radiation and duration of exposure. A study presented at an annual meeting of Radiology Society of North America (RSNA) observed that high-risk women exposed before age 20 or with five or more exposures were 2.5 times more likely to develop breast cancer than high-risk women not exposed to low-dose radiation [9]. This limits the mammography as a frequent screening modality.
3. *Fear and pain:* To get proper mammograms, breast region should be compressed. An approximate of 15–20 pounds of pressure is applied on the breast region to image. Due to high compression involved, sometimes it might also lead to rupture of tumor. Many surveys described this as painful screening method that subjects would like to avoid [10].
4. *Privacy:* Apart from pain and fear of radiation, it is reported in Ref. [11] that nearly 38% among women from different ethnic groups and with more than 60% among South Asian countries like India and Pakistan do not go for screening due to embarrassment of disrobing.

Thermography overcomes the above issues and enables more people to go for screening. It can work on women of all age groups. It is a non-contact, non-invasive modality with passive infrared measurement, which does not involve any radiation, hence a safe screening method. Since the thermal images can essentially be captured from a laptop connected to the thermal camera, it is also extremely privacy aware.

Among other modalities, clinical breast exam can detect tumors only once they are large enough to be palpable and result in many false positives. Effective use of sono-mammography (ultrasound) for cancer detection requires location of the lump. Hence, ultrasound is best used as a correlation modality. Once a lump is detected either through mammography or thermography or clinical breast examination, ultrasound will be very useful to reconfirm malignancy or not.

4. Biological explanation

Cancer cells release nitric oxide [12, 13] into the blood and lead to alteration in microcirculation. This nitric oxide coupled with aggressiveness of cancer to grow increases the blood circulation by dilating the vessels and leads to creation of new blood vessels (neo-angiogenesis) and dormant vessel recruiting. Experimentally, Folkman [14, 15] observed this dependency of tumor growth with angiogenesis by implanting tumour cells in mice. Large volume of blood flow in these vessels connected to tumor makes them hotter when compared to normal blood vessels. This large flow distorts the vessel structure, and vessels become dilated as well as elongated, causing the increase in the dimension of vessel caliber and length [16, 17]. This elongation combined with the large flow deviates the vessel structure from normal vessels by making them more tortuous due to formation of bends [18–20]. In fact, it is experimentally evident that this high tortuosity is observed much before angiogenesis [18].

In addition, it has been empirically observed that tumor temperature is higher than the neighboring temperatures with the help of contact temperature measurements. In Ref. [21], Gautherie claimed that this high heat is due to high metabolic activity at tumor location. Hence, this region appears brighter and hotter in thermographic images when compared to surroundings. It is also observed that tumor temperature is warmer compared to the blood vessels feeding the tumor region [21]. Aggressiveness of cancer cells makes the boundary of tumor irregular as they break the boundary formed by basal laminas to invade the neighboring tissues [19, 20]. This is not seen in case of benign tumors whose cells behave similar to normal cells. This makes the benign tumor boundaries regular.

The size of tumor indicates the stage of cancer and largely affects the survival rate. A survey conducted by Narod [2] observed drastic decrease in survival rate with increase in tumor size. Early detection of cancer increases the chances of survival. Thermography outperforms other modalities when it comes to early detection. Changes such as vasodilation, neo-angiogenesis and high tortuosity of blood vessels which are found in initial stages of cancer result in thermal impressions and hence can be detected in thermography [15–19]. These might not be observed in other modalities which depend upon detecting architectural distortions that appear only when tumor is sufficiently grown. A study by Gautherie and Gros [3] over 58,000 patients for 12 years showed that thermography detected breast cancer five years earlier in around 400 patients than mammography and ultrasonography.

Abnormality in thermogram is not the sole criterion for malignancy. Increase in heat pattern might even be observed due to hormonal response, lactation and presence of benign tumors such as fibrocystic and fibroadenoma. However, these non-malignant conditions have different projections in the thermographic image when compared to malignant tumors. Unlike in malignant breasts where there is asymmetrical heat map, heat response is mostly symmetrical across the two breasts with high hormonal response. Estrogen released during hormonal activity produces nitric oxide that causes increase in heat and vessel dilation [12]. Similar activity happens in the case of lactating mothers except that a little asymmetry in heat map is seen due to uneven lactation in both breasts. There is an increase in heat signature even in benign cases such as fibrocystic and fibroadenoma [21, 22]. In contrast to malignant tumors, these cells are not aggressive and behave similar to normal cells [19, 23]. Other than these cases, abnormal heat pattern leading to vasodilation and angiogenesis can also occur during inflammation caused by infection or wound healing [12, 14]. Though these abnormalities are formed, they have distinct features compared to malignancy that can be distinguished.

Some recent explorations have shown that thermography can even help in prognosis. Since the increase of temperature in malignant tumors is primarily due to the release of nitric oxide, which is caused due to hormonal activity, the temperature distribution on the breasts also provides signals on the hormonal receptor status of malignant tumors. Zore et al. [9] have studied the effect of hormone receptor status of malignant tumors on thermograph through a quantitative analysis of average or maximum temperatures of the tumor, the mirror tumor site and the breasts. While no statistically significant difference was found in the overall temperature distribution in breasts with hormone receptors being positive or negative, they report a significant difference in average and maximum tumor temperature measurements. Another computer-aided study [24] reported an accuracy of more than 80% for automated estimation of hormonal receptor status of malignant tumors. This shows the potential of a non-invasive way of predicting the hormone receptor status of malignancies through thermal imaging, before going through Immuno-Histo-Chemistry (IHC) analysis on the tumor samples after surgery.

5. Protocols for capturing thermal images

A standard imaging protocol has to be followed for any modality to make it a repeatable and operator agnostic procedure that can reduce subjectivity and errors in image capture. Likewise, a set of instructions has to be followed in thermography as well [25, 26].

Most importantly, before capturing the images, patient must be cooled for minimum period of 10–15 min in a room maintained at a temperature of 16-22 °C. This helps in attaining thermal equilibrium with the surrounding environment [25]. Cooling is mandatory as it helps in removal of extraneous heat caused due to external reasons such as tight clothing, apparel and friction from a hand bag or outside temperature. Cooling also helps in enhancing the temperature pattern of tumorous regions compared to non-tumourous regions [27–30]. It is observed that normal tissue reacts quickly to external cooling, whereas malignant reacts slowly, making it appear hotter compared to rest of the breast region. For quick cooling of images, cold challenge can be used where patient hands are immersed in cold water causing the regulation of body temperature with sympathetic stimulus [30].

When it comes to capturing the actual thermal images, imaging protocols can be categorized into discrete and continuous imaging protocols.

Discrete imaging protocols: These protocols are interested in specific set of static fixed views. The basic views which are observed in most discrete protocols include frontal view (0°), oblique views (±30°) and lateral views (±90°). Some variations of different protocols in the way of the mentioned views are captured, such as (a) seated position, (b) supine position, (c) standing position and (d) combinations of {a,b,c}. Subset of mentioned views/changing the angle of views/ adding more view angles are also being used in some studies.

A tumor has less effect with cooling compared to normal tissues whose heat signatures decrease drastically [28, 30]. To study the nature of cancer cells further, some protocols include the above combinations of different views after cooling the breasts. Some protocols consider only fully cooled breasts, while some capture the breast image before and after cooling and analyze the thermal patterns of the cooled breast and uncooled breasts [31].

Continuous imaging protocols: Continuous imaging protocols capture videos of the breast as they are cooled, instead of static images. These protocols are not as popular as discrete due to the large processing time needed to analyze. However, much larger information can be captured in a video. For example, tumorous regions do not cool as fast as rest of the tissues.

6. Advances in thermal cameras

Medical thermography is also benefiting from the rapid advancement in the quality of thermal imaging too. Temperature capture has evolved from a complicated probe-based method to a camera-based registration.

Over the years, improvements in silicon technology have made a huge impact on the technology used in IR detectors. Many use cases of thermal imaging are evolving in biomedical, transport, energy and environmental applications, and they have been the key business driver for this growth, as well. **Figure 1** depicts the history of development of infrared sensors, which is very well described in Ref. [32]. The real breakthroughs were focal plane arrays and bi-dimensional arrays improving spatial resolution and thermal sensitivity.

Broadly, infrared cameras can be divided into cooled and uncooled detectors. Cooled thermal cameras have infrared detectors integrated with cryocoolers and enable measurement of very low temperatures as well as very high resolution and improved sensitivity as thermally-induced noise is reduced. However, cooled cameras are expensive and may be needed only for applications that require very high resolution and high sensitivity.

Microbolometer focal plane arrays (FPAs) have tremendously modified the way of image capture by allowing an array of sensors at the focal plane of lens to detect the LWIR wavelengths [32, 33]. This integration has led to the development of uncooled infrared detectors that are typically small, handheld and also restricted the need for expensive cooling techniques. The current uncooled cameras work on the principle of change in resistance or voltage or current due to the emitted infrared radiation. The resolution is direct function of number of pixels in the microbolometer array per unit area. With the advances in silicon technology, these digital infrared uncooled cameras have massively transformed from a low resolution to high resolution of 640 × 480 pixels to 1024 × 768 pixels or more. The current cameras also have improved the sensors to obtain a thermal sensitivity and accuracy error of at most 20 mK and 1°C respectively. To detect the infrared radiation, vanadium oxide (VOx) and amorphous silicon are common materials in microbolometer [32].

The lens is costly compared to lens found in normal video-shoot cameras, since normal glass cannot be used to make the lens due to its property of blocking LWIR radiation and reflecting the LWIR incident on the lens. Hence, Germanium (Ge), Chalcogenide glass, Zinc Selenide (ZnSe) and Zinc Sulfide (ZnS) that are LWIR-transmissive are used for the lens preparation.

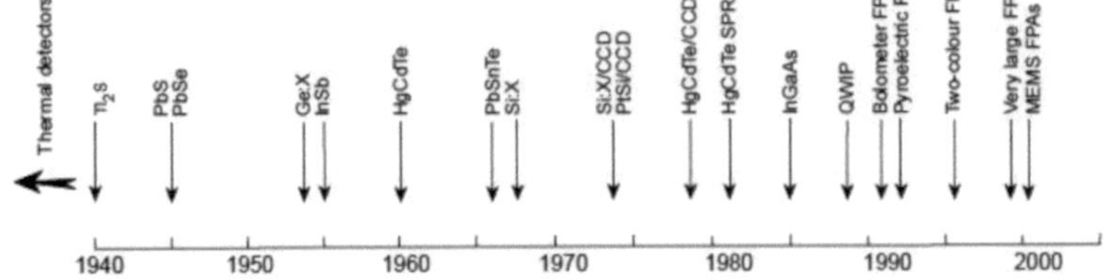

Figure 1. Advances in thermal sensor technology (reproduced from Ref. [32]).

These uncooled cameras have also reduced the cost and heavy maintenance that would be needed for the cooled detectors. Some popular camera models used for medical purposes are shown in **Figure 2**. Today, FLIR, Fluke and Meditherm are thermal camera vendors preferred by thermographers for medical thermography as many of these camera models are already FDA-certified for tele-thermology.

6.1. Visual interpretation of thermal images

There are different protocols followed by thermographers for analyzing and interpreting thermal images, especially for breast cancer screening. Most of this work in creating the protocols have taken place in the 1970s and 1980s, such as the Marseille protocol [13–15], Hobbins protocol [30], Gautherie protocol [21], Hoekstra protocol [34] and, more recently, with newer thermal cameras, the Villa Marie protocol [12]. An attempt to obtain an agreement of different experienced thermographers was also made in 1975 to provide a consistent set of observations to be noted [17].

All of these protocols give different thermographic category ratings of four to five levels, starting from normal to highly suspicious of malignancy. Multiple criteria are noted, using both vascular and non-vascular observations. These criteria are generally qualitative rather than quantitative. The visual interpretation necessitates heuristic rules to combine these observations to determine a thermographic category. Some protocols assign numbers to each observation and combine them using a mathematical function for categorization. This also shows the need for experience and proper training for thermographic interpretation.

Regardless of the variations across protocols, these criteria can be broadly classified into vascular and non-vascular criteria, with some generality in these criteria, as follows:

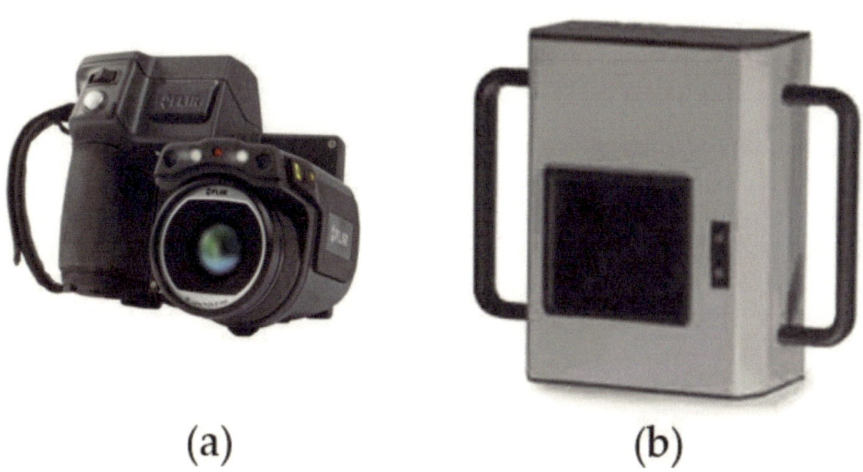

Figure 2. Two thermal camera models from different vendors (a) FLIR T650SC (b) Meditherm IRIS 2000.

Non-vascular criteria:

1. Focal increase in temperature by a fixed interval, e.g., 1, 2, 3°C
2. Global increase in temperature compared to the contralateral breast by, say, 1.5°C
3. Regional increase in temperature, including specific quadrants
4. Differences in temperature between contralateral regions or between different quadrants/ regions in the same side
5. Abnormal location of focal increase including areolar regions or along edges/bulges
6. Abnormal physical observations: bulging/size variation, retraction

Vascular criteria:

1. Vascular asymmetry
2. Vascular anarchy, including tortuous or serpentine or loops or clusters or bifurcations
3. Increased vascular density
4. Abnormal directions of clusters of vessels, such as vertical, horizontal
5. Number of vessels
6. Caliber of vessels
7. Abnormal location of vascularity and avascularity

The general interpretation from these protocols is that with few and mild abnormal findings, the categorization is toward normal and likely benign. With increased abnormality, the observations tend toward increased suspicion of malignancy. Another important point to note is that benign diseases also exhibit some abnormal thermal vascular/non-vascular criteria [30]. The diagnosis for benign conditions is made by follow-up of thermography over a few months, by which time the abnormal thermal findings change or reduce or disappear.

Due to these multiple diverse metrics used by practitioners and no standardized way of interpretation across different expert thermographers, the thermological interpretation becomes very subjective and many times results in high false positives. Many efforts are therefore underway to remove subjectivity using computer-aided diagnostic methods—some of which are described later in this chapter.

7. Clinical validations

Thermography is not a new technique for breast cancer screening. Its presence has been there since 1960 [26]. There have been many longitudinal and clinical trials performed to show its efficacy. In 1982, FDA approved thermography as an adjunct modality for breast cancer screening. **Table 1** lists out the studies that has been done to show the potential of thermography. This technique is undervalued due to the difficulty in interpreting the thermograms with naked eye. The interpretation varies from observer to observer and needs high expertise to correctly validate the diagnosis result, limiting to few thermographers. With advent of technology, in both hardware and software, automated analysis of thermograms is emerging to obtain high sensitivity and specificity.

Studies	Subjects	Follow-up	Results	Comments
Gershon-Cohen [41], 1967	1924	No follow-up	Sensitivity—91.6% Specificity—92.4%	
Stark and Way [42], 1974	4621	No follow-up	Sensitivity—98.3% Specificity—93.5%	–
Spitalier [43, 44], 1982	61,000	10-Year period	Sensitivity—89% Specificity—89%	They reported that thermography was the first alarm in 60% cancer cases and stated that abnormal thermogram represents
Haberman [45], 1980	39,802	3-Year period	Sensitivity—85% Specificity—70%	30% of cancers showed their initial signs in thermography compared with traditional screening
Gros and Gautherie [3, 21, 46, 47], 1980	85,000	5-Year period for 58,000 patients	Sensitivity—90% Specificity—88%	Out of 1245 women that showed -ve signs with traditional screening in their first visit, more than 33% have got cancer in this 5-year period
Jones [48], 1983	70,000	No follow-up	Sensitivity—87% Specificity—85%	
Parisky [37], 2003	769	No follow-up	Sensitivity—97%	
Rassiwala [49], 2014	1008	No follow-up	Sensitivity—97.6% Specificity—99.2%	

Table 1. List of large-scale studies.

8. Advances in software technology

As seen in the clinical validation, the sensitivity observed with visual analysis is acceptable, but specificity is lower than desired with visual interpretation. Further, visual observations and heuristic categorization are subject to human error and variation through subjective interpretation. To solve these problems, there are automated and semiautomated approaches for diagnostics [35]. We review some of the software tools available from companies who are intending to provide a replicable method of interpreting thermal images.

We review the technology used in three such software tools from Niramai health, Total vision and Mammo vision. All these approaches use static images obtained after cooling the subject with discrete imaging protocols.

8.1. Visualization tools for thermal interpretation

Given that a thermologist has to look at five colored images, where the temperature differences between neighboring regions need to be identified by minute color variations, interpretation of thermal breast images is a huge cognitive overload and very error prone. So, software tools that aid in visualization and capturing of the observations about thermal patterns are becoming available.

Total vision software from Med-hot.com gives an excellent visualization of the thermal images and additional support for a thermographer to systematically look for specific abnormal thermal pattern alongside a rule-based decision-making support to simplify the interpretation process. However, it does not have any automation of the diagnosis.

Mammo vision [31] is a semi-automated tool that tries to identify the non-vascular abnormal thermal patterns during dynamic thermography with cold challenge. It considers 10 images in total, 5 images before cooling and 5 images after cooling, for the analysis. An elliptical grid is used to approximate breast region, and it automatically extracts the lateral symmetry, isothermia in each quadrant, areolar temperature, nipple temperature, temperature decrease with cooling and hotspot parameter. Additionally, the clinician can manually identify the vascularity in the breast by looking at grayscale thermal image, which is then used by the tool to categorize the subjects into five groups. The tool defines assessment criteria called Breast Infrared Assessment System (BIRAS) with which they categorize the images into five groups with BIRAS 1 being low risk and BIRAS 5 being high risk.

8.2. Use of sophisticated computer-aided diagnostics

Use of sophisticated artificial intelligence algorithms for enabling automatic diagnosis or clinical interpretation guidance is most needed to reduce subjectivity in interpretation [37]. Niramai Thermalytix software is one such advanced software tool with a technology that enables end-to-end fully automated approach for the diagnosis [38–40]. The Niramai tool uses complex computer algorithms for the following five key aspects of automated diagnostics.

1. Autotagging

Since one single view may not be sufficient to capture tumor region in different parts of the breast region, multiple views are taken. Typically, there are five thermal images in multiple views that are captured; one of the common mistakes done by clinicians is to name the image wrongly. It is observed that many a times humans are confused with classification of right and left sides of breast in the image correctly and resulting in improper tagging of lateral and oblique views. Hence, Niramai software provides an automated tagging support. This reduces the error in naming or false tagging, which in turn would have resulted in other errors such as segmentation error and misclassification of subjects. Their software automatically tags the views based on the body border curvature and body area.

http://dx.doi.org/10.5772/intechopen.69198

2. Detecting the region of interest

The thermal image is captured with the patient sitting about three feet from the camera. This captures the thermal signature of the top part of body of the subject starting from neck region. A tool like Niramai that does automatic analysis of breast cancer has to accurately crop the region of interest (ROI), namely the breast tissue region. For this, Niramai tool removes inframammary fold, axilla, sternum and thyroid regions that are usually warm regions and might unnecessarily cause false positives. Additional heuristic based on the shape of body gives accurate segmentation of the ROI as shown in **Figure 3**. There is considerable research in the detection of ROI for single view [35], and tools that provide manual support through freehand segmentation and adjustable and draggable ellipse that the clinician can use mark the region of interest. Niramai software automatically detects the breast region using a polygon approximation of region that makes it easier for a clinician to edit, if needed.

3. Tumor localization

Once the region of interest for analysis is determined, next technical challenge is to accurately identify the exact location of an abnormality or a lesion. This usually means detecting regions having warm and hot temperature pixels in the image and analyzing the heat pattern around the same. The heat patterns found in the thermal images are then analyzed for specific tumor properties. Tumor-specific patterns include multiple important thermal patterns or features that typically help in discriminating malignancy versus benign conditions [38].

Symmetry plays a significant role in detecting whether a hot patch is abnormal. So, a subset of the ROI showing a significant increase in temperature as compared to the neighboring areas and contralateral sides is identified. In NIRAMAI, two varieties of abnormal regions

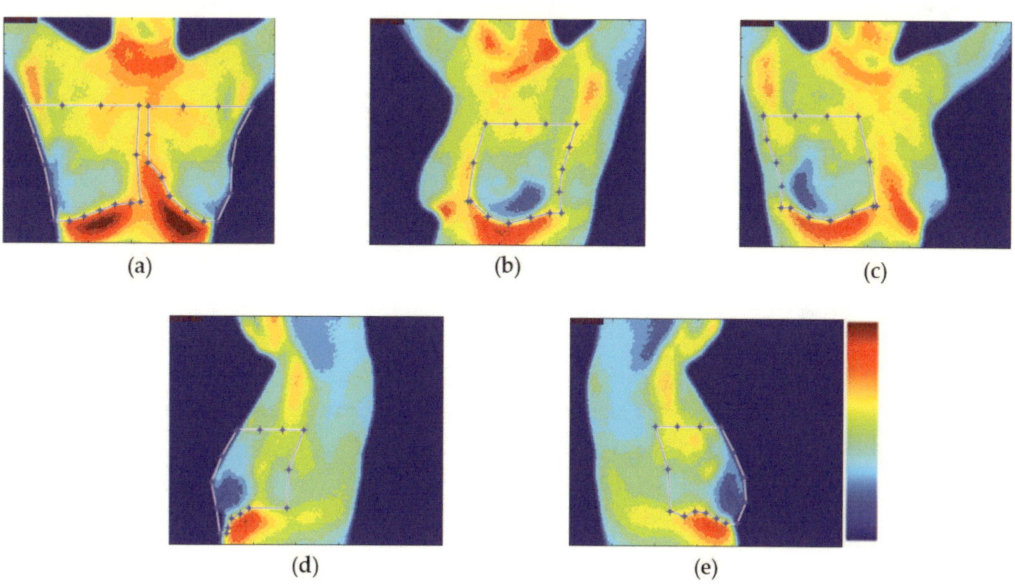

Figure 3. Results of automated segmentation in different views. (a) Frontal (b) Left Oblique (c) Right Oblique (d) Left Lateral (e) Right Lateral.

are extracted, hot-spots and warm-spots, based on the degree of their thermal response. This categorization helps to increase sensitivity with low thermal response tumors without increasing the false positives. Hot-spots correspond to high-temperature regions segmented using a combination of temperature-based thresholds. Warm-spots correspond to slightly lower temperature regions as compared to hot-spots with a change in parameters. One way of categorizing the same is using the modes and maximum temperature values, as shown in Eqs. (1) and (2).

$$T_a = T_{overallmax} - \mathrm{T} \quad (1)$$

$$T_b = \Gamma + \mathrm{P}(T_{overallmax} - \Gamma) \quad (2)$$

In above equations, Γ refers to the mean of the modes of the ROI temperature histograms in all views, and $T_{\text{overallmax}}$ represents the overall maximum temperature in all views. (P, T) are parameters chosen depending on the dataset.

Niramai tool detects hot-spots and warm-spots in each view of the subject. The best views of hot-spots and warm-spots are defined as the view in which the normalized size of the detected abnormal regions with respect to the ROI is maximum. **Figure 4** shows some sample subject images with their corresponding hotspots identified by NIRAMAI tool. From the detected hot-spots in multiple views, the hot-spots and warm spots corresponding to the best view are usually used to extract core features. Since symmetry places an important role, features are also extracted using the best view and its contralateral side view.

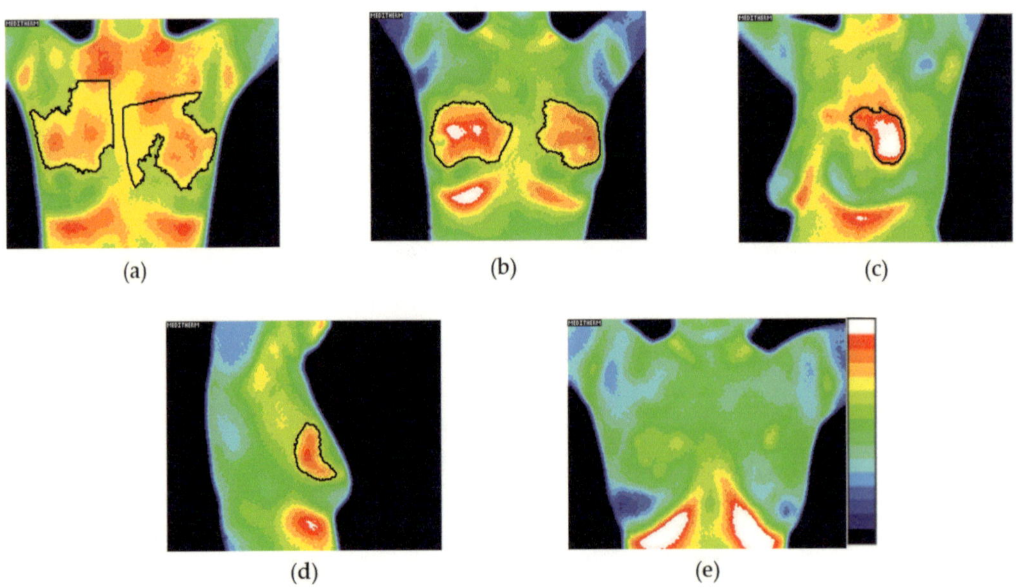

Figure 4. Sample subject images for (a) hormone-sensitive tissues showing warm-spots, (b) lactating case showing warm-spots, (c) malignant case showing hot-spots, (d) benign case showing warm-spots and (e) normal case.

4. Feature extraction

Once the hot- and warm-spots showing potential lesion is detected, three high-level properties of the lesion are extracted. These are boundary features, thermal symmetry and temperature distribution.

Malignant tumor cells are aggressive in nature, which makes them to invade surrounding tissues by rupturing through the boundary formed by basal laminas [19]. This makes the boundary irregular for malignant cases compared to non-malignant and benign cases which behave similar to normal cells.

In the case of malignant tumors, benign tumors, inflammation or wound-healing cases, an increase in temperature in the abnormal regions is observed. This leads to a difference in thermal heat patterns compared to the contralateral breasts. However, similarity in thermal heat patterns is seen for normal, hormonal, lactating conditions [12, 22, 36] due to the presence of similar hormone-sensitive tissues in both the breasts. This property is captured by including symmetrical features.

Finally, the mean temperature difference between the detected abnormal region and the remaining region of interest is calculated to get the relative increase in temperature compared to the neighboring region. In addition, many other temperature parameters of the abnormal region can be used for analysis.

5. Automated classification

Computer algorithms based on artificial intelligence and machine learning are making huge inroads in automated diagnostics [38]. Many methods of supervised classification are being developed where a small group of patient data is used to train a probabilistic model that represents the decision criteria based on the extracted features. A simple such classifier is a random forest that is able to identify the significant discriminatory features and learns a combination of the features and feature groups that helps decide on malignancy subjects. Other classifiers include support vector machines, Kmeans classifiers and deep learning.

9. Conclusions

In the recent years, use of Information Technology in healthcare diagnostics is proving to be very effective in improving efficiency and quality of care. Thermography is highly suited for breast cancer screening owing to its ability to detect cancer much earlier than any other modality, patient safety and privacy. The complexity and subjectivity in interpretation of thermal imaging has been a major deterrent in wide acceptance of the usage of thermography. Use of computer-aided diagnostics for automated thermography interpretation is just round the corner. With software support, thermal analysis and interpretation can be more efficient, effective and non-subjective. This chapter described some of the recent developments in both the hardware and the software of a thermographic solution that shows great promise that breast thermography will be a mainstream cancer screening modality very soon.

Author details

Siva Teja Kakileti[1], Geetha Manjunath[1*], Himanshu Madhu[1] and Hadonahalli Venkataramanappa Ramprakash[2]

*Address all correspondence to: geetha@niramai.com

1 NIRAMAI Health Analytix Pvt Ltd, Bangalore, India

2 Central Diagnostics Research Foundation, Bangalore, India

References

[1] Nickson C, Kavanagh AM. Tumor size at detection according to different measures of mammographic breast density. Journal of Medical Screening. 2009;**16**(3):140-146. DOI: 10.1258/jms.2009.009054

[2] Narod SA. Tumor size predicts long-term survival among women with lymph node-positive breast cancer. Current Oncology. 2012;**19**(5):249-253

[3] Gautherie M, Gros CM. Breast thermography and cancer risk prediction. Cancer. 1980;**45**(1):51-56. DOI: 10.1002/cncr.2820450110

[4] American College of Clinical Thermology. ACCT Approved Thermography Clinics [Internet]. Available from: http://www.thermologyonline.org/Breast/breast_thermography_clinics.htm [Accessed: March 25, 2017]

[5] Kolb TM, Lichy J, Newhouse JH. Comparison of the performance of screening mammography, physical examination, and breast US and evaluation of factors that influence them: An analysis of 27 825 patient evaluations. Radiology. 2002;**25**(1). DOI: 10.1148/radiol.2251011667

[6] Skaane P. Studies comparing screen-film mammography and full-field digital mammography in breast cancer screening: Updated review. Acta Radiology. 2009;**50**(1):3-14. DOI: 10.1080/02841850802563269

[7] Svahn TM, Chakraborty DP, Ikeda D, Zackrisson S, Do Y, Mattsson S, Andersson I. Breast tomosynthesis and digital mammography: A comparison of diagnostic accuracy. The British Journal of Radiology. 2017;**85**(1019):e1074–e1082. DOI: 10.1259/bjr/53282892

[8] Ginsburg OM, Martin LJ, Boyd NF. Mammographic density, lobular involution, and risk of breast cancer. British Journal of Cancer. 2008;**99**(9):1369-1374. DOI: 10.1038/sj.bjc.6604635

[9] Zore Z, Boras I, Stanec M, Orešić T, Zore IF. Influence of hormonal status on thermography findings in breast cancer. Acta Clinica Croatica. 2013;**52**(1):35-42

[10] Collins K, Winslow M, Reed MW, Walters SJ, Robinson T, Madan J, Green T, Cocker H, Wyld L. The views of older women towards mammographic screening: A qualitative and quantitative study. British Journal of Cancer. 2010;**102**(10):1461-1467

[11] Forbes LJL, Atkins L, Thurnham A, Layburn J, Haste F, Ramirez AJ. Breast cancer awareness and barriers to symptomatic presentation among women from different ethnic groups in East London. British Journal of Cancer. 2011;**105**(10):1474-1479. DOI: 10.1038/bjc.2011.406

[12] Kennedy DA, Lee T, Seely D. A comparative review of thermography as a breast cancer screening technique. Integrative Cancer Therapies. 2009;**8**(1):9-16. DOI: 10.1177/1534735408326171

[13] Thomsen LL, Miles DW, Happerfield L, Bobrow LG, Knowles RG, Moncada S. Nitric oxide synthase activity in human breast cancer. British Journal of Cancer. 1995;**72**(1):41

[14] Folkman J. What is the evidence that tumors are angiogenesis dependent? Cancer Spectrum Knowledge Environment. 1990;**82**(1):4-6

[15] Folkman J. Tumor angiogenesis: Therapeutic implications. New England Journal of Medicine. 1971;**285**(21):1182-1186

[16] Konerding MA, Malkusch W, Klapthor B, van Ackern C, Fait E, Hill SA, Parkins C, Chaplin DJ, Presta M, Denekamp J. Evidence for characteristic vascular patterns in solid tumors: Quantitative studies using corrosion casts. British Journal of Cancer. 1999;**80**(5-6):724

[17] Goel S, Duda DG, Xu L, Munn LL, Boucher Y, Fukumura D, Jain RK. Normalization of the vasculature for treatment of cancer and other diseases. Physiological Reviews. 2011;**91**(3):1071-1121

[18] Li C-Y, Shan S, Huang Q, Braun RD, Lanzen J, Hu K, Lin P, Dewhirst MW. Initial stages of tumor cell-induced angiogenesis: Evaluation via skin window chambers in rodent models. Journal of the National Cancer Institute. 2000;**92**(2):143-147

[19] Baish JW, Jain RK. Fractals and cancer. Cancer Research. 2000;**60**(14):3683-3688

[20] Bullitt E, Zeng D, Gerig G, Aylward S, Joshi S, Smith JK, Lin W, Ewend MG. Vessel tortuosity and brain tumor malignancy: A blinded study. Academic Radiology. 2005;**12**(10):1232-1240

[21] Gautherie M. Thermobiological assessment of benign and malignant breast diseases. American Journal of Obstetrics and Gynecology. 1983;**147**(8):861-869

[22] Keyserlingk JR, Ahlgren PD, Yu E, Belliveau N, Yassa M. Functional infrared imaging of the breast. IEEE Engineering in Medicine and Biology Magazine. 2000;**19**(3):30-41

[23] Harvey L, et al. Cancer. In: Harvey L, editor. Molecular Cell Biology. 7th ed. New York: W.H. Freeman and Co.; 2013. pp. 1113-1148

[24] Kakileti S, Venkataramani K, Madhu H. Automatic determination of hormone receptor status in breast cancer using thermography. In: 19th International Conference on Medical Image Computing and Computer-Assisted Intervention—MICCAI. Vol. 9900. Springer; 2016. DOI: 10.1007/978-3-319-46720-7_74

[25] Ring EFJ, Ammer K. The technique of infrared imaging in medicine. Thermology International. 2000;**10**(1):7-14

[26] Amalu WC, Hobbins WB, Head JF, Elliot RL. Infrared imaging of the breast. In: Diakides M, Bronzino JD, Peterson DR, editors. Medical Infrared Imaging: Principles and Practices. CRC Press; Taylor & Francis Group, Boca Raton, Florida. 2012. pp. 10.1-10.22. DOI: 10.1201/b12938-11

[27] Gautherie M. Thermopathology of breast cancer: Measurement and analysis of in vivo temperature and blood flow. Annals of the New York Academy of Sciences. 1980; **335**(1):383-415

[28] Laaperi E, Laaperi AL, Strakowska M, Wiecek B, Przymusiala P. Cold provocation improves breast cancer detection with IR thermography: A pilot study. Thermology International. 2012;**22**(4):152-156

[29] Ohashi Y, Uchida I. Applying dynamic thermography in the diagnosis of breast cancer. IEEE Engineering in Medicine and Biology Magazine. 2000;**19**(3):42-51

[30] Hobbins WB. Thermography of the breast—A skin organ. In: Thermal Assessment of Breast Health. proceedings of an international conference held in Washington, DC, USA, July 20-24, 1983. pp. 40-48

[31] Berz R, Schulte-Uebbing C. MammoVision (infrared breast thermography) compared to X-ray mammography and ultrasonography. In: Diakides M, Bronzino JD, Peterson DR, editors. Medical Infrared Imaging: Principles and Practices. CRC Press; 2012. pp. 12.1-12.12. DOI: 10.1201/b12938-13

[32] Rogalski A. Infrared detectors: Status and trends. Progress in Quantum Electronics. 2003;**27**(2):59-210

[33] Corsi C. Infrared: A key technology for security systems. Advances in Optical Technologies. 2012;**2012**. DOI: 10.1155/2012/838752

[34] Carmeliet P, Jain RK. Angiogenesis in cancer and other diseases. Nature. 2000;**407** (6801):249-257

[35] Borchartt TB, Conci A, Lima RCF, Resmini R, Sanchez A. Breast thermography from an image processing viewpoint: A survey. Signal Processing. 2010;**93**(10):2785-2803

[36] Gautherie M. Improved system for the objective evaluation of breast thermograms. Progress in Clinical and Biological Research. 1982;**107**:897

[37] Parisky YR, Sardi A, Hamm R, Hughes K, Esserman L, Rust S, Callahan K. Efficacy of computerized infrared imaging analysis to evaluate mammographically suspicious lesions. American Journal of Roentgenology. 2003;**180**(1):263-269. DOI: 10.2214/ajr.180.1.1800263

[38] Madhu H, Kakileti ST, Venkataramani K, Jabbireddy S. Extraction of medically interpretable features for classification of malignancy in breast thermography. In: 2016 IEEE 38th Annual International Conference of the Engineering in Medicine and Biology

Society (EMBC); August; Orlando, Florida. IEEE; 2016. pp. 1062-1065. DOI: 10.1109/EMBC.2016.7590886

[39] Kakileti ST, Venkataramani K. Automated blood vessel extraction in two-dimensional breast thermography. In: 2016 IEEE International Conference on Image Processing (ICIP); September; Phoenix, Arizona. IEEE; 2016. pp. 380-384. DOI: 10.1109/ICIP.2016.7532383

[40] Venkataramani K, Mestha LK, Ramachandra L, Prasad SS, Kumar V, Raja PJ. Semi-automated breast cancer tumor detection with thermographic video imaging. In: 37th Annual International Conference of the IEEE Engineering in Medicine and Biology Society (EMBC). IEEE; 2015. pp. 2022-2025

[41] Gershon-Cohen J, Haberman-Brueschke JA, Brueschke EE. Medical thermography: A summary of current status. Radiologic clinics of North America. 1965;**3**(3):403

[42] Stark, Agnes M, Way S. The screening of well women for the early detection of breast cancer using clinical examination with thermography and mammography. Cancer. 1974;**33**(6):1671-1679. DOI: 10.1002/1097-0142(197406)33:6<1671::AID-CNCR2820330630>3.0.CO;2-4

[43] Spitalier H, Giraud D, et al. Does infrared thermography truly have a role in present day breast cancer management?. In: Liss AR, editor. Biomedical Thermology. New York: 1982. pp. 269-278.

[44] Amalric R, Giraud D, Altschuler C, Amalric F, Spitalier JM, Brandone H, Ayme Y, Gardiol AA. Does infrared thermography truly have a role in present-day breast cancer management?. Progress in Clinical and Biological Research. 1981;**107**:269-278

[45] Haberman, JoAnn D, Love, Francis TJ, John E. Screening a rural population for breast cancer using thermography and physical examination techniques: Methods and results-A preliminary report. Annals of the New York Academy of Sciences. 1980;**335**(1):492-500. DOI: 10.1111/j.1749-6632.1980.tb50774.x

[46] Sciarra J. Breast cancer: Strategies for early detection. In: Thermal Assessment of Breast Health (Proceedings of the International Conference on Thermal Assessment of Breast Health); MTP Press LTD; 1983. pp. 117-129

[47] Louis K, Walter J, Gautherie M. Long-term assessment of breast cancer risk by thermal imaging. In: Liss AR, editor. Biomedical Thermology; New York: 1982. pp. 279-301

[48] Jones CH. Thermography of the female breast. Diagnosis of Breast Disease. Baltimore: University Park Press; 1983. pp. 214-234

[49] Rassiwala M, Mathur P, Mathur R, Farid K, Shukla S, Gupta PK, Jain B. Evaluation of digital infra-red thermal imaging as an adjunctive screening method for breast carcinoma: A pilot study. International Journal of Surgery. 2014;**12**(12):1439-1443. DOI: http://dx.doi.org/10.1016/j.ijsu.2014.10.010

Chapter 6

Incorporating Breast Asymmetry Studies into CADx Systems

José María Celaya Padilla,
Cesar Humberto Guzmán Valdivia,
Jorge Issac Galván Tejada, Carlos Eric Galván Tejada,
Hamurabi Gamboa Rosales,
Juan Rubén Delgado Contreras,
Antonio Martinez-Torteya, Roberto Olivera Reyna,
Jorge Roberto Manjarrez Sánchez,
Francisco Javier Martinez Ruiz, Idalia Garza-Veloz,
Margarita L. Martinez-Fierro, Victor Treviño and
Jose Gerardo Tamez-Peña

Additional information is available at the end of the chapter

http://dx.doi.org/10.5772/intechopen.69526

Abstract

Breast cancer is one of the global leading causes of death among women, and an early detection is of uttermost importance to reduce mortality rates. Screening mammograms, in which radiologists rely only on their eyesight, are one of the most used early detection methods. However, characteristics, such as the asymmetry between breasts, a feature that could be very difficult to visually quantize, is key to breast cancer detection. Due to the highly heterogeneous and deformable structure of the breast itself, incorporating asymmetry measurements into an automated detection system is still a challenge. In this study, we proposed the use of a bilateral registration algorithm as an effective way to automatically measure mirror asymmetry. Furthermore, this information was fed to a machine learning algorithm to improve the accuracy of the model. In this study, 449 subjects (197 with calcifications, 207 with masses, and 45 healthy subjects) from a public database were used to train and evaluate the proposed methodology. Using this procedure, we were able to independently identify subjects with calcifications (accuracy = 0.825, AUC = 0.882) and masses (accuracy = 0.698, AUC = 0.807) from healthy subjects.

Keywords: breast cancer, asymmetry, bilateral registration, CAD

1. Introduction

Cancer is one of the leading causes of death worldwide. In 2008, nearly 13% (7.6 million) of all deaths were cancer related. Among all types of cancer, lung, liver, colon, breast, and cervical are the most frequent ones. Recent studies predict 13.1 million cancer deaths for 2030 [1]. Among women, breast cancer is the deadliest type of cancer. Nearly 1.8% of all worldwide deaths are breast cancer related [2].

Till today, there is no cure for breast cancer, and since the trigger to develop any type of cancer is still a mystery, there is not an effective way to prevent the occurrence. Early detection of breast cancer plays a key role in a positive prognosis. There are several imaging technologies that might be used by specialists for the early detection of breast cancer, such as magnetic resonance imaging, ultrasound, and X-ray mammogram. The last technique is the primary tool used to diagnose and detect breast cancer worldwide, and it has been proved to be the best cost-effective tool to diagnose the disease [3].

In clinical practice, mammography allows for the detection of early signs of tumors before they become apparent [3]. Common signs of early cancer inside the breast tissue are microcalcifications, architectural distortions, and masses [4]. During the screening procedure, radiologists use those signs to generate a standardized evaluation of the risk of cancer in a given patient, called Breast Imaging-Reporting and Data System (BI-RADS). This report helps oncologists to decide a course of action among women at risk of developing breast cancer [5].

The broad use of mammogram has driven the development of computer-aided detection (CADe) and computer-aided diagnosis (CADx) systems. While both approaches aim to assist radiologists to detect and diagnose breast cancer as early as possible, CADx systems are used as a second opinion [6] and CADe ones aim to improve visualization of the lesions (with up to 35% improvement in detection rate [7]). However, although it has been shown that CADe systems have helped radiologists to better interpret findings [8], it has also been demonstrated that in some cases they may make interpreting the images more difficult, reducing the accuracy of early cancer detection [7]. Furthermore, these systems also may increase the workload of the radiologists [8].

A typical CADe system, whose workflow is shown in **Figure 1**, consists of two algorithms applied sequentially, one to detect suspicious regions or regions of interest (ROI), and one to refine such regions. The former includes the preprocessing of the images, segmentation of

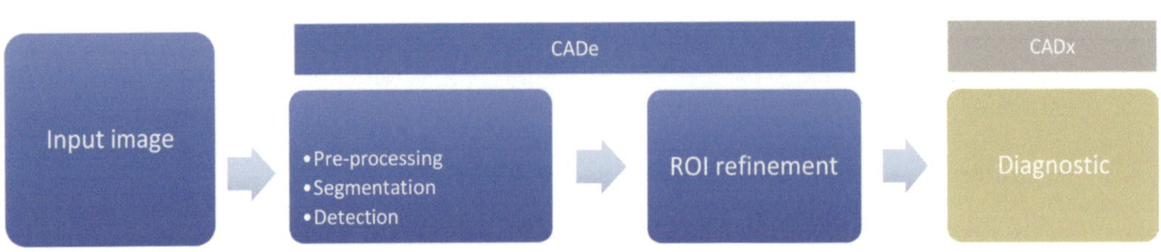

Figure 1. Typical workflow of a CADe/CAD*x* system, adapted from Chen g et al. [13].

the breast tissue, and the detection of the ROI itself. The latter process is performed to reduce the number of false positives [8], and usually relies on machine learning techniques [9–11]. Lastly, the results are presented to the radiologist, highlighting in the original mammography the regions that the analysis deemed highly suspicious. As seen in the same image, CADx systems follow the same workflow as CADe ones. However, besides highlighting areas of higher risk to the radiologist, additional algorithms are used to analyze each ROI and generate a computer-based diagnosis. It is important to mention that, currently, few CADe and CADx commercial systems have been approved by the Food and Drug Administration of the United States of America [12].

Many methodologies used by CADx systems analyze only one breast, or even just a subregion of the breast, at a time. That is, they evaluate the left and right breasts as independent objects, unlike radiologists, who analyze images of both breasts simultaneously to evaluate their asymmetry. Radiologists do so because asymmetry is related to early signs of breast cancer (i.e. parenchymal distortion, bright spots, masses, etc.) [14, 15] and it may be used to reduce the rate of false positive detection of masses [16, 17]. Asymmetry can refer to either a longitudinal study, where current and prior mammograms are compared, or a bilateral study, where differences between the left and right breast are analyzed.

A few CADx systems have already tried to incorporate asymmetry studies to enhance diagnosis [14, 18–20]. Some researchers have studied the use of a feature-based asymmetry analysis, where the mammograms are processed individually and the differences between the individual analyses are used as a mean to quantify asymmetry [21]. This approach has also been used to characterize risk factors, such as breast density, and predict near-term breast cancer [14].

Another method that evaluates asymmetry, this one trying to mimic the approach used by radiologists, is the mammogram subtraction. In this approach, differences between mammograms are enhanced by performing a rigid registration (alignment) of the images. However, this methodology was originally employed only in longitudinal studies [22], comparing the same breast at two different times, since the highly heterogeneous and deformable tissue of the breast has hindered the inclusion of subtraction approaches in bilateral asymmetry studies [19].

Miller et al. [23] proposed a technique for the detection of bilateral symmetry using a semi-automated texture-based procedure that segments the glandular tissue, measuring the shape between views, and thus detecting the occurrence of asymmetries. The algorithm obtained an accuracy of 0.867 on a validation dataset of 30 screening mammogram pairs. Later, Miller et al. [24] presented a method for the detection of bilateral asymmetry based on measures of shape, topology, and distribution of brightness. This method was tested on 104 mammogram pairs, yielding a classification accuracy of 0.74.

Lau et al. [25] proposed a method for the detection of breast tumors that extracted measures of brightness, roughness, and directionality, and was based on localized asymmetry. This method was evaluated using 10 pairs of mammograms where asymmetry was a significant factor in the radiologist's diagnosis. A sensitivity of 0.92 was obtained, with 4.9 false positives per mammogram. However, the alignment was tuned manually using control points.

Ferrari et al. [26] characterized asymmetry as variations in oriented textural patterns, obtained using directional filtering with Gabor wavelets at different orientations and scales. Using a database with 80 images resulted in a classification accuracy of up to 0.744.

Rodriguez-Rojas et al. [21] presented a CADx system targeted to detect high-risk cancer patients. To do so, automated breast tissue segmentations were performed on 200 Mexican subjects labeled as either low- or high-risk according to their BI-RADS score. Then, 50 features were extracted, and bilateral differences between mammograms were defined by subtracting corresponding features in both mammograms. Finally, a genetic algorithm selected a predictive combination of features. Using this methodology, they were able to classify low-risk and high-risk cases with an area under the receiver operating characteristic (ROC) curve (AUC) of 0.88 on a 150-fold cross-validation set. The features included in the model were associated with the differences in signal distribution and tissue shape.

In summary, and as presented, most asymmetry detection methods are either feature-based, rely on simple bilateral subtraction techniques [14, 27], or depend on an ROI provided by a radiologist [24, 25]. Thus, in order to efficiently measure asymmetry, a better and automatic registration must be performed [28]. To do so, alignment has been improved by using the nipple as a reference point [29] and by co-registering both breasts using a robust point matching approach [22]. Nevertheless, none of those works include a fully automated bilateral registration. In this chapter, a methodology that incorporates an automatic asymmetry analysis with both a feature-based and a pixel-wise bilateral subtraction into a CADx system is presented.

2. Methodology

The proposed methodology follows the CADx workflow presented in the previous section. However, asymmetry measurements are used to aid in the diagnosis. To obtain such measurements, two additional stages are incorporated into the workflow: registration and pixel-wise subtraction. Additionally, a series of image transformations are incorporated to enhance different characteristics of the breast in the mammograms. This work is based on and follows previous efforts [30–32].

Figure 2 shows how the bilateral asymmetry information was incorporated into the CADx system. Briefly, soft tissue is first segmented, the image of the left breast is then registered to its right counterpart and a bilateral subtraction of the co-registered images is performed;

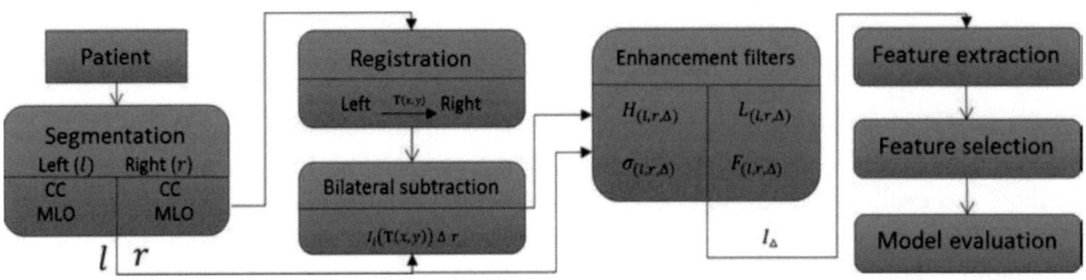

Figure 2. Workflow of the proposed methodology.

images are then filtered and features are extracted; a multivariate model is selected using a train set; and finally, the model is evaluated on a validation set. A detailed explanation of each stage is presented in the following sections.

2.1. Materials

A total of 1796 digitalized film mammograms from 449 different subjects were used. From those, 45 were classified as healthy subjects (HS) (mean age of 59.3 and standard deviation (SD) of 9.8 years), 197 as subjects with malignant calcifications (CS) (mean age of 58 and SD of 10.9 years), and 207 as subjects with malignant masses (MS) (mean age of 64.1 and SD of 10.1 years). Each subject had the four standard mammograms taken, namely, left and right craniocaudal (CC), and left and right mediolateral oblique (MLO) projections.

In order to avoid problems associated with intra-scanner variability [17, 22, 33], all mammograms in this study were obtained from the Howtek dataset of the Digital Database for Screening Mammography public database [34], in which all mammograms were digitalized using a Howtek 960 scanner using a sampling rate of 43.5 micrometers per pixel and a 12-bit depth.

2.2. Segmentation

Segmentation, also called categorization by computer vision definitions, allows delimiting one or several parts of a given image assigning one class label (e.g. bone, muscle, fat, skin, calcification, and mass). This process is defined by the division or segmentation of the image into several homogeneous regions disjointed from their surroundings. A commonly used automatic segmentation of the breast tissue is based on the estimation of the background noise. For this study, an initial segmentation mask was created by estimating the background noise in the image and discarding all pixels below five standard deviations of the noise level. Then, holes were removed by applying closing morphological operations with a 3 × 3 supporting region, as described by Eq. (1):

$$S(A) = (A(x,y) \oplus B(x,y)) \ominus B(x,y) \quad (1)$$

where $\oplus$ and $\ominus$ are the grayscale dilation and erosion morphological operations, respectively. B (x, y) is a 3 × 3 structural element. $A\ (x, y)$ is the image being segmented and $S\ (A)$ is the resulting segmentation of the $A\ (x, y)$ image. The largest connected region is used as the segmentation mask while all other high-intensity regions are removed from the images. **Figure 3** shows an example of the results of the segmentation procedure.

2.3. Registration

Image registration can be defined as the intensity and spatial mapping between two images [35]. Given two input images F and M, image registration can be expressed as $R' = g[T(F)]$, where T is a spatial transformation function, g an intensity transformation function, and R' the registered image. The transformation function is not always necessary; a lookup table can be used to pinpoint intensities. A visual example of image registration is presented in **Figure 4**, where an image M is being registered to match image F.

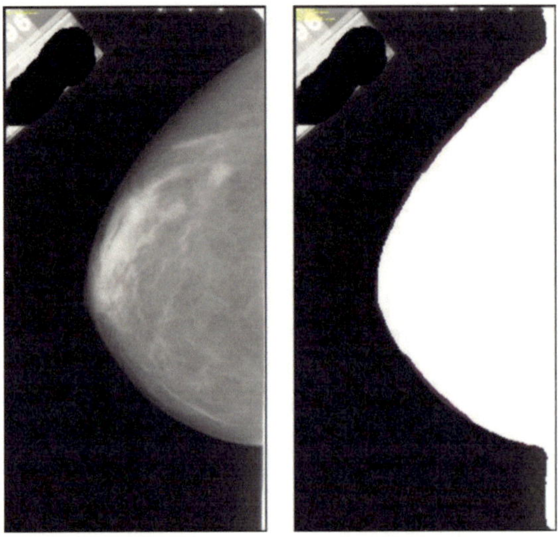

Figure 3. Segmentation of breast tissue. The image on the left is the original CC mammogram and the image on the right shows the superimposed segmentation mask in white (image from Ref. [32]).

Image registration has been widely used in medical applications [28, 36, 37]. However, the soft nature of the breast tissue makes them highly deformable, and rigid registration procedures, in which only rotation, translation, and scaling functions are used, are not sufficient. Therefore, nonrigid registration methods are necessary [38, 39]. There are many approaches to deal with medical imaging registration, the most recent comparison of algorithms based on a retrospective evaluation was published by West et al. [40], but it was constrained to do intra-patient rigid registration. Also recently, Diez et al. [28] and Celaya-Padilla et al. [30] compared registration algorithms with breast images as a source, and both concluded that the B-Splines approach was the most consistent.

Breast image registration based on a B-Splines transformation is defined as follows: given two input images (F = target image, M = image being registered), M is deformed by modifying a mesh of control points following a maximization of a similarity measure based on steepest descent gradient [6, 15]. The deformed image is compared to F using a similarity metric. If the images are similar enough, the process stops. Otherwise, the process reiterates.

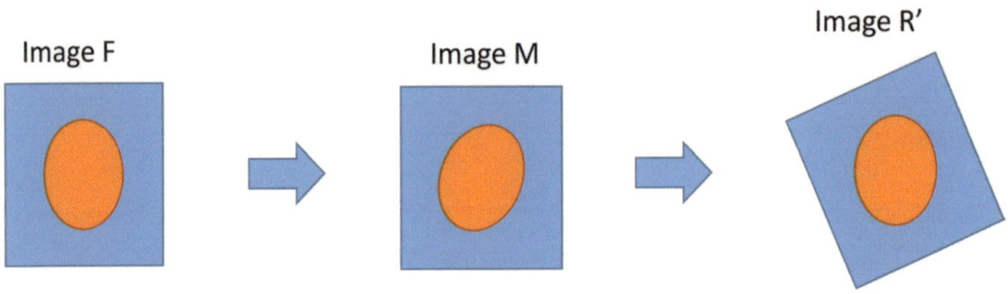

Figure 4. Basic example of an image registration procedure. F is the target image, M is the image to be registered, and R' is the registered image.

Figure 5 shows a multi-resolution pyramid approach [41] for the B-Spline implementation. There, the images are first registered using low-resolution images, the B-Spline transformation parameters are moved into the next higher resolution and parameter optimization is run again, and so on. This often avoids issues with local minima in the parameter search space and reduces computational time [15].

For this study, the image to be registered was first horizontally flipped. Then, both the moving image and the target image were resampled into a lower resolution image. Next, the pyramids for the multi-resolution were generated. Afterwards, the registration process detailed in **Figure 5** was carried out. And finally, the original moving image was deformed using the final parameters of the registration. For this implementation, mutual information [39] was used as the similarity metric. In **Figure 6**, the checkerboard of an example result from the B-Spline registration procedure is presented. There, it can be seen that the registered image was successfully aligned with its counterpart.

2.4. Image subtraction

Once the images were co-registered, a pixel-wise absolute difference was computed between the left and right images, as defined by Eq. (2) as follows:

$$I_{\triangle}(x,y) = \left| I_r(x,y) - I_l(T(x,y)) \right| \tag{2}$$

where $I_r(x, y)$ represents the right image, $I_l(\mathbf{T}(x, y))$ represents the left image registered to the right image space, and $I_{\Delta}(x, y)$ represents the map of absolute differences. **Figure 7** shows an example of the differential image for two given input images.

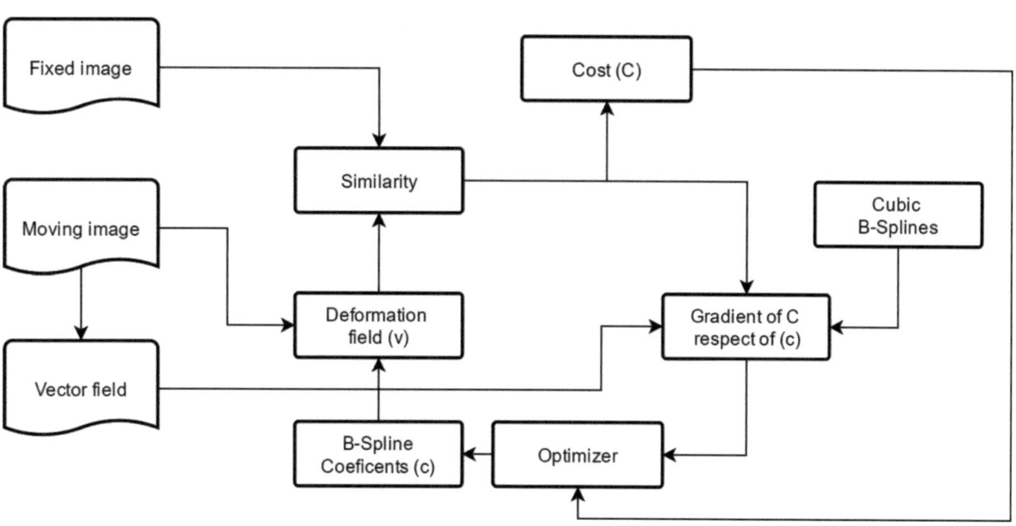

Figure 5. B-Spline registration typical framework.

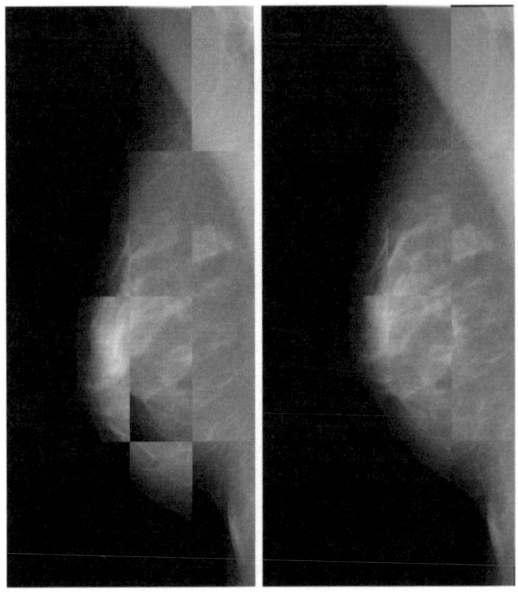

Figure 6. Checkerboard comparison of images *pre* and *post* B-Spline registration. The image in the left shows a comparison between a left and horizontally flipped right breast before registration, and the right image shows the results of the registering process.

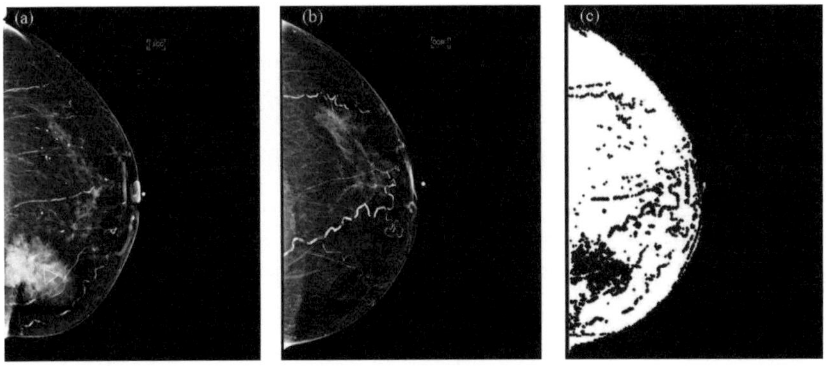

Figure 7. Image subtraction example. Left: unaltered CC view of left breast, middle: horizontally flipped CC view of right breast, and right: color map of the subtraction image I_Δ. White and black pixels inside the breast tissue represent small and large intensity differences, respectively.

2.5. Image enhancement

To study the appearance of the architectural distortions, two enhancing filters were applied to the images: a morphological high-frequency enhancement filter (*H*) designed to enhance fiber-like tissues, and a Laplacian of Gaussian filter (*L*) that enhances high-frequency patterns inside the breast tissue. Additionally, since the texture between normal and abnormal tissues is different [42], two texture maps were created. The first map computed the local standard deviation (σ) of the mammograms, and the second map computed the local fractal dimension (F). All image processing was implemented in C++ using Insight Segmentation and Registration Toolkit (ITK) libraries for image manipulation following previous efforts [32, 43].

2.6. Feature extraction

There are several features that may be quantified when aiming to detect early signs of cancer. For this analysis, 43 features were extracted from each image. These features can be grouped in three main categories: shape (i.e. area, perimeter, compactness, elongation, region centroid, region scatter), signal (i.e. mean, median, energy, variance, standard deviation, dynamic range, z mean, entropy, skewness, kurtosis, z range, fraction greater than z deviations, fraction lower than z deviations, value at fraction, 5% trimmed mean, 5% trimmed standard deviation, 5% trimmed z *Mean*), and morphology (i.e. total signal, signal centroid, signal scatter, and signal surface). Details of the full feature extraction procedure can be found in Ref. [32].

The enhancement filters and texture maps presented in Section 2.5 were applied to the four screening mammograms (i.e. left and right CC, and left and right MLO) and to the two bilateral subtraction images (CC and MLO), yielding a set of 15 images for both the CC and the MLO views: I_r, I_l, I_Δ, H_r, H_l, H_Δ, L_r, L_l, L_Δ, σ_r, σ_l, σ_Δ, F_r, F_l, and F_Δ, where I is the raw image, H, L, σ, and F are the enhanced images described in Section 2.5, and r, l, and Δ, stand for the right, left, and bilateral subtraction images, respectively. Features were then extracted from this set of images. Additionally, to study the feature-based asymmetry analysis, the average and absolute difference of each left-right pair of measurements was also analyzed, resulting in 860 additional features, resulting in a total of 2150 features per subject.

2.7. Feature selection

The first step of the feature selection process consisted discarding highly correlated to avoid redundancy. For any pair of features with a Spearman correlation coefficient larger than 0.96, one feature was randomly selected to be kept, and the other removed from the selection. The dataset was normalized using the empirical distribution of the healthy subjects and a z-normalization was performed using the rank-based inverse normal transformation [44].

In order to select the most accurate and compact set of features from each dataset, the least absolute shrinkage and selection operator (LASSO) method was used [45]. The shrinkage and selection method minimizes the sum of squared errors and penalizes the regression coefficients, as described by Eq. (3) as follows:

$$\hat{\beta}^{\text{lasso}} = \operatorname{argmin} \sum_{i=1}^{N} \left(y_i - \beta_0 - \sum_{j=1}^{p} x_{ij} \beta_j \right)^2 \text{ subject to:} \sum_{j=1}^{p} |\beta| \le t \tag{3}$$

Given a set of input measurements $x_1 \ldots x_n$ and an outcome y, the lasso method fits a linear model where x_i is the covariate vector for the ith case and y_i is the outcome, t is a tuning parameter that determines the amount of regularization, and N is the number of cases.

The multivariate search was performed using a class balanced data sample of 100 subjects for training and the remaining subjects as a blind test set. The models were calibrated using a leave-one-out cross-validation strategy, training the models at every split using $N-1$ subjects and evaluating the model using the remaining subjects [46]. The final reported performance was obtained by applying the final model gathered on the training stage and evaluating it in the blind test set.

3. Results

A total of 1796 mammograms were successfully segmented. The image sets of nine subjects had to be removed from the experiment due to problems with the registration process, six were from MS, two from CS, and one from HS. All the remaining subjects were included in the subsequent stages of the analysis. The 2150 extracted features were filtered by the correlation process, removing 826 features.

Table 1 shows the features that were selected for each model: the CS versus HS ($n = 12$), and the MS versus HS ($n = 16$). The former achieved an accuracy of 0.825 with an AUC of 0.882 and the latter an accuracy of 0.698 with an AUC of 0.807. **Figure 8** shows the ROC curves for both the models.

	CS versus HS			MS versus HS		
#	View	Image	Feature	View	Image	Feature
1	CC	H_Δ	27	CC	L_Δ	40
2	CC	F_Δ	13	CC	I_r	29
3	CC	I_r	29	CC	L_l	40
4	CC	H_l	29	CC	F_r	6
5	CC	H_l	6	MLO	H_l	11
6	MLO	I_l	28	CC	$L_{\Delta avg}$	29
7	MLO	H_l	11	CC	$I_{\Delta s}$	28
8	MLO	H_l	21	CC	$\sigma_{\Delta s}$	38
9	CC	$I_{\Delta s}$	28	CC	$F_{\Delta avg}$	12
10	CC	$\sigma_{\Delta s}$	38	MLO	$I_{\Delta s}$	40
11	MLO	$L_{\Delta avg}$	27	MLO	$I_{\Delta s}$	28
12	CC	H_Δ	27	MLO	$I_{\Delta s}$	29
13				MLO	$H_{\Delta s}$	31
14				MLO	$H_{\Delta s}$	7
15				MLO	$L_{\Delta avg}$	39
16				MLO	$L_{\Delta avg}$	27

Note: Features are grouped by dataset, symmetric features are denoted with:

$$I_{\Delta avg} = \frac{I_r + I_l}{2}, H_{\Delta avg} = \frac{H_r + H_l}{2}, \mathrm{L}_{\Delta avg} = \frac{L_r + L_l}{2}, \sigma_{\Delta avg} = \frac{\sigma_r + \sigma_l}{2}, F_{\Delta avg} = \frac{\sigma_r + \sigma_l}{2},$$

$$\mathrm{I}_{\Delta s} = |I_r - I_l|, H_{\Delta s} = |H_r - H_l|, \mathrm{L}_{\Delta s} = |H_r - H_l|, \sigma_{\Delta s} = |H_r - H_l|, F_{\Delta s} = |H_r - H_l|.$$

Table 1. Features of the proposed models.

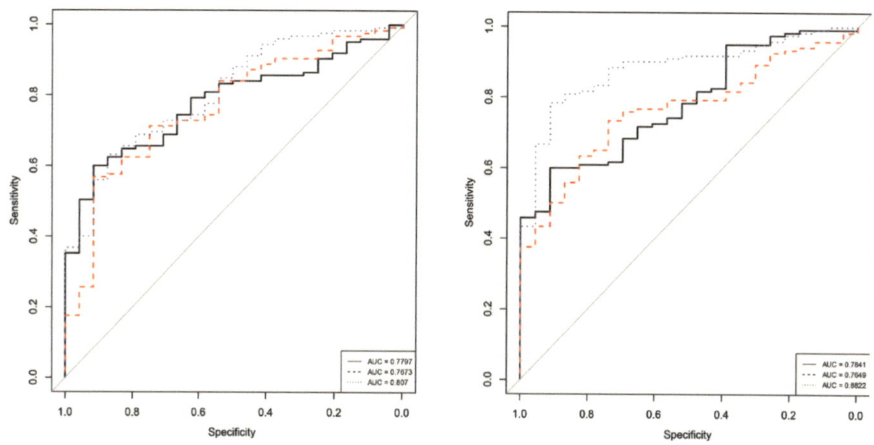

Figure 8. ROC curves for the classification models. Left: MS versus HS, right: CS versus HS. The dashed line represents the model with the features from only the difference images, the solid line the one with features from only the raw images, and the dotted line the one with the features from all images (from Ref. [32]).

4. Discussion

The proposed methodology is fully automated and does not require manual intervention as previous proposals [16, 17]. Although the approach is similar to others [22], we did not attempt to remove the pectoral muscle from the segmentation mask, since the presence of abnormal axillary lymph in this area is an indicator of occult breast carcinoma [47]. However, from the computational point of view, the feature extraction process may be affected if the region processed is not well focused [48].

The proposed registration process achieved a good performance having only 2.0% of the subjects that had to be discarded due to registration issues. This performance is remarkable when considering the amount of deformation undergoing in a mammography procedure. The B-spline deformation is an improvement over rigid or affine co-registration methods [33]. The advantage of the deformable registration has been recognized as a key element in breast analysis and has been successfully used in longitudinal studies [22]. Regarding digital subtraction, the differences in the X-ray projection, and image acquisition and digitizing artifacts may affect the detection of asymmetric patterns. Our results indicate that even in the presence of registration artifacts, the digital subtraction added information that was successfully incorporated during the feature selection process.

The B-Spline transformation algorithm, proposed for the bilateral mammogram registration presented, shows a clear improvement after the registration. Due to lack of temporal mammograms, temporal registration was not tested. Nevertheless, the methodology could be implemented in such task. However, the temporal registration should be re-optimized using a new set of parameters.

The enhanced images and texture maps enriched the feature set providing a four-fold increase in extracting features per patient, which were also incorporated in the final classification models. Regarding symmetry, the strategy of exploring bilateral symmetry has been explored by other researchers where a series of features (signal, texture, breast density, etc.) were computed from each mammogram and the absolute difference between both breasts was obtained to measure breast tissue asymmetry, and used it to predict the likelihood of developing cancer [19]. We extended this idea by registering the left and right images using a deformable transformation, which increased the number of features per patient by 25%.

This study shows that healthy subjects, subjects with calcifications, and subjects with masses can accurately be classified through models generated via mammography registration and a feature selection methodology. The analysis of the feature selection strategy demonstrated that even when using a different approach for the feature selection strategy, the proposed methodology achieved similar results as the previously presented ones. Therefore, we can say that the methodology is robust to the feature selection strategy.

The methodology demonstrated that the image subtraction of registered images generates information that aids in the identification of subjects with lesions, such as malignant masses and calcifications. The methodology also incorporated the use of feature-based asymmetry into the CADx system. The combination performance achieved has the potential to be used to queue cases with a high chance of malignant findings, or may have the practical use of triaging mammograms in developing countries where there is a deficiency of expert readers.

Author details

José María Celaya Padilla[1*], Cesar Humberto Guzmán Valdivia[1], Jorge Issac Galván Tejada[2], Carlos Eric Galván Tejada[2], Hamurabi Gamboa Rosales[2], Juan Rubén Delgado Contreras[3], Antonio Martinez-Torteya[4], Roberto Olivera Reyna[2], Jorge Roberto Manjarrez Sánchez[5], Francisco Javier Martinez Ruiz[2], Idalia Garza-Veloz[6], Margarita L. Martinez-Fierro[6], Victor Treviño[7] and Jose Gerardo Tamez-Peña[7]

*Address all correspondence to: jose.celaya@uaz.edu.mx

1 Autonomous University of Zacatecas/ CONACyT – Universidad Autónoma de Zacatecas (CONACyT – UAZ), Jardín Juarez, Centro, Zacatecas, Zacatecas, Mexico

2 Electric Engineering Department, Autonomous University of Zacatecas (UAZ), Jardín Juarez, Centro, Zacatecas, Zacatecas, Mexico

3 Superior Technical Institute of Zacatecas South (ITSZaS), Las lomitas, Tlaltenango, Zacatecas, Mexico

4 Engineering Department, Monterrey University (UdeM), Morones Prieto Pte, Jesús M. Garza, San Pedro Garza García, Nuevo Leon, Mexico

5 Computer Engineering Systems Department, Superior Technical Institute of Jerez (ITSJ) Libramiento Fresnillo-Tepetongo, Fracc. Los Cardos, Jerez de García Salinas, Zacatecas, Mexico

6 Health Sciences Department ,Human Medical School, Autonomous University of Zacatecas (UAZ), Jardín Juarez, Centro, Zacatecas, Zacatecas, Mexico

7 Bioinformatic group, Medical School, Monterrey Institute of Technology (ITESM), Eugenio Garza Sada, Monterrey, Nuevo Leon, Mexico

References

[1] World-Health. Cancer Fact sheet No. 297 [Internet]. 2015. Available from: http://www.who.int/mediacentre/factsheets/fs297/en/index.html [Accessed: 09/02/2015]

[2] DeSantis C, Ma J, Bryan L, Jemal A. Breast cancer statistics, 2013. CA: A Cancer Journal for Clinicians. 2014;**64**(1):52-62

[3] Ng K, Muttarak M. Advances in mammography have improved early detection of breast cancer. Honk Kong College or Radiologist. 2003;**6**(3):126-131

[4] Chan H-P, et al. Computer-aided classification of mammographic masses and normal tissue: Linear discriminant analysis in texture feature space. Physics in Medicine and Biology. 1995;**40**(5):857-876

[5] D'orsi C, Bassett L, Berg W, Feig S, Jackson V, Kopans D. Breast Imaging Reporting and Data System: ACR BI-RADS-Mammography. Reston: American College of Radiology (ACR); 2003

[6] Doi K. Current status and future potential of computer-aided diagnosis in medical imaging. The British Journal of Radiology. 2005;**78**(1):S3-S19

[7] Sampat MP, Markey MK, Bovik AC, et al. Computer-aided detection and diagnosis in mammography. Handbook of Image and Video Processing. 2005;**2**(1):1195-1217

[8] Dromain C, Boyer B, Ferre R, Canale S, Delaloge S, Balleyguier C. Computed-aided diagnosis (CAD) in the detection of breast cancer. European Journal of Radiology. 2013;**82**(3):417-423

[9] Ramos-Pollán R, et al. Discovering mammography-based machine learning classifiers for breast cancer diagnosis. Journal of Medical Systems. 2012;**36**(4):2259-2269

[10] Li M, Zhou Z-H. Improve computer-aided diagnosis with machine learning techniques using undiagnosed samples. IEEE Transactions on Systems, Man and Cybernetics, Part A: Systems and Humans. 2007;**37**(6):1088-1098

[11] Doi K. Computer-aided diagnosis in medical imaging: historical review, current status and future potential. Computerized Medical Imaging and Graphics. 2007;**31**(4-5):198-211

[12] Eadie LH, Taylor P, Gibson AP. A systematic review of computer-assisted diagnosis in diagnostic cancer imaging. European Journal of Radiology. 2012;**81**(1):e70-e76

[13] Cheng H-D, Cai X, Chen X, Hu L, Lou X. Computer-aided detection and classification of microcalcifications in mammograms: A survey. Pattern Recognition. 2003;**36**(12):2967-2991

[14] Zheng B, Sumkin JH, Zuley ML, Wang X, Klym AH, Gur D. Bilateral mammographic density asymmetry and breast cancer risk: A preliminary assessment. European Journal of Radiology. 2012;**81**(11):3222-3228

[15] Scutt D, Lancaster GA, Manning JT. Breast asymmetry and predisposition to breast cancer. Breast Cancer Research. 2006;**8**(2):R14

[16] Giger ML, Yin FF, Vyborny CJ. Comparison of bilateral-subtraction and single-image processing techniques in the computerized detection of mammographic masses. Investigative Radiology. 1993;**28**(6):473-481

[17] Yin FF, Giger ML, Doi K, Metz CE, Vyborny CJ, Schmidt RA. Computerized detection of masses in digital mammograms: Analysis of bilateral subtraction images. Medical Physics. 1991;**18**(5):955-963

[18] Tan M, Zheng B, Ramalingam P, Gur D. Prediction of near-term breast cancer risk based on bilateral mammographic feature asymmetry. Academic Rradiology. 2013;**20**(12):1542-1550

[19] Wang X, Lederman D, Tan J, Wang XH, Zheng B. Computerized prediction of risk for developing breast cancer based on bilateral mammographic breast tissue asymmetry. Medical Engineering & Physics. 2011;**33**(8):934-942

[20] Wang X, Lederman D, Tan J, Wang XH, Zheng B. Computerized detection of breast tissue asymmetry depicted on bilateral mammograms: A preliminary study of breast risk stratification. Academic Radiology. 2010;**17**(10):1234-1241

[21] Rodriguez-Rojas J, Garza-Montemayor M, Trevino-Alvarado V, Tamez-Pena JG. Predictive features of breast cancer on Mexican screening mammography patients. In: Spie Medical Imaging. International Society for Optics and Photonics; Florida, USA. 2013, pp. 867023-867023-9

[22] Martí R, Díez Y, Oliver A, Tortajada M, Zwiggelaar R, Lladó X. Detecting abnormal mammographic cases in temporal studies using image registration features. In: Breast Imaging. Springer; Gifu, Japan. 2014. pp. 612-619

[23] Miller P, Astley SM. Detection of breast asymmetry using anatomical features. In: IS&T/SPIE's Symposium on Electronic Imaging: Science and Technology. International Society for Optics and Photonics; Los Ángeles California, USA. 1993. pp. 433-442

[24] Miller P, Astley S. Automated detection of breast asymmetry using anatomical features. State of the Art in Digital Mammographic Image Analysis, Series in Machine Perception and Artificial Intelligence. 1994;**9**:247-261

[25] Lau TK, Bischof WF. Automated detection of breast tumors using the asymmetry approach. Computers and Biomedical Research. 1991;**24**(3):273-295

[26] Ferrari RJ, Rangayyan RM, Desautels JL, Frère AF. Analysis of asymmetry in mammograms via directional filtering with Gabor wavelets. IEEE Transactions on Medical Imaging. 2001;**20**(9):953-964

[27] Suri JS, Rangayyan RM. Recent Advances in Breast Imaging, Mammography, and Computer-Aided Diagnosis of Breast Cancer. SPIE press; Washington, USA. 2006. pp. 488-525

[28] Diez Y, et al. Revisiting intensity-based image registration applied to mammography. IEEE Transactions on Information Technology in Biomedicine. 2011;**15**(5):716-725

[29] Mendez AJ, Tahoces PG, Lado MJ, Souto M, Correa JL, Vidal JJ. Computer-aided diagnosis: Automatic detection of malignant masses in digitized mammograms. Medical Physics. 1998;**25**:957

[30] Celaya-Padilla JM, Rodriguez-Rojas J, Trevino V, Tamez-Pena JG. Local image registration a comparison for bilateral registration mammography. In: Presented at the International Seminar on Medical Image Processing and Analysis; Mexico, DF; 2013

[31] Celaya-Padilla JM, Rodriguez-Rojas J, Galván-Tejada JI, Martínez-Torteya A, Treviño V, Tamez-Peña JG. Bilateral image subtraction features for multivariate automated classification of breast cancer risk. In: SPIE Medical Imaging. International Society for Optics and Photonics; San Diego, CA, USA. 2014. pp. 90351T-90351T-7

[32] Celaya-Padilla J, Martinez-Torteya A, Rodriguez-Rojas J, Galvan-Tejada J, Treviño V, Tamez-Peña J. Bilateral image subtraction and multivariate models for the automated triaging of screening mammograms. BioMed Research International. 2015;**2015**:1-12

[33] Yin FF, Giger ML, Doi K, Vyborny CJ, Schmidt RA. Computerized detection of masses in digital mammograms: Automated alignment of breast images and its effect on bilateral-subtraction technique. Medical Physics. 1994;**21**(3):445-452

[34] Heath M, Bowyer K, Kopans D, Moore R, Kegelmeyer P. The digital database for screening mammography. In Proceedings of the 5th International Workshop on Digital Mammography. San Diego, CA, USA. 2000. pp. 212-218

[35] Guo Y, Suri J, Sivaramakrishna R. Image registration for breast imaging: A review. In: 27th Annual International Conference of the IEEE Engineering in Medicine and Biology Society, 2005. IEEE-EMBS 2005. IEEE; Toronto, Canada. 2006. pp. 3379-3382

[36] Marias K, Behrenbruch C, Parbhoo S, Seifalian A, Brady M. A registration framework for the comparison of mammogram sequences. IEEE Transactions on Medical Imaging. 2005;**24**(6):782-790

[37] Kok-Wiles SL, Brady M, Highnam R. Comparing mammogram pairs for the detection of lesions. In Digital Mammography. Springer; Nijmegen, Netherlands. 1998. pp. 103-110

[38] Hill DL, Hawkes DJ. Across-modality registration using intensity-based cost functions. In Handbook of Medical Imaging. Academic Press, Inc; Orlando, FL, USA. 2000. pp. 537-553

[39] Mattes D, Haynor DR, Vesselle H, Lewellyn TK, Eubank W. Nonrigid multimodality image registration. In: Medical Imaging 2001. International Society for Optics and Photonics; San Diego, CA, USA. 2001. pp. 1609-1620

[40] West J, et al. Comparison and evaluation of retrospective intermodality brain image registration techniques. Journal of Computer Assisted Tomography. 1997;**21**(4):554-568

[41] Rosenfeld A. Multiresolution Image Processing and Aanalysis. Springer Science & Business Media; Heidelberg, Germany. 2013

[42] Rangayyan RM, Banik S, Desautels JL. Computer-aided detection of architectural distortion in prior mammograms of interval cancer. Journal of Digital Imaging. 2010;**23**(5):611-631

[43] Ibanez L, Schroeder W, Ng L, Cates J. The ITK Software Guide. Kitware; New York, USA. 2003

[44] Beasley TM, Erickson S, Allison DB. Rank-based inverse normal transformations are increasingly used, but are they merited? Behavior Genetics. 2009;**39**(5):580-595

[45] Tibshirani R. Regression shrinkage and selection via the lasso. Journal of the Royal Statistical Society. Series B (Methodological). 1996;**58**:267-288

[46] Friedman J, Hastie T, Tibshirani R, Regularization Paths for Generalized Linear Models via Coordinate Descent. Journal of Statistical Software, Innsbruck, Austria, 2010;**33**(1):1-22

[47] Ganesan K, Acharya UR, Chua KC, Min LC, Abraham KT. Pectoral muscle segmentation: A review. Computer Methods and Programs in Biomedicine. 2013;**110**(1):48-57

[48] Raba D, Oliver A, Martí J, Peracaula M, Espunya J. Breast segmentation with pectoral muscle suppression on digital mammograms. In: Pattern Recognition and Image Analysis. Springer; Berlin, Heidelberg, Germany. 2005. pp. 471-478

Chapter 7

Initial Clinical Evaluation of Observer Performance Using a Tablet Computer with a 4K High-Resolution Display for Detection of Breast Cancer by Digital Mammography

Ryusuke Murakami, Nachiko Uchiyama,
Hitomi Tani and Shinichiro Kumita

Additional information is available at the end of the chapter

http://dx.doi.org/10.5772/intechopen.69074

Abstract

Purpose: To compare observer performance using medical-purpose 5-megapixel liquid crystal display monitors (5-MP LCDs) and a tablet PC with a 4K high-resolution display for detection of breast cancer by digital mammography. **Materials and methods:** Mammograms from 40 patients with primary breast cancer (18 mass, 16 microcalcifications, 3 artificial distortions, and 3 focal asymmetries) and 60 control patients were consecutively collected. Four experienced radiologists assessed 100 mammograms to rate using the BI-RADS lexicon. The BI-RADS assessments were subjected to receiver operating characteristic (ROC) curve analysis. Also, the observers assessed the image quality in terms of brightness, contrast, sharpness, and noise using 5-step Likert scale. **Results:** The average under the curve (AUC) values for use of the 5-MP LCDs and 4K monitors were 0.921 and 0.936; the difference between them was small and not significant. In terms of image quality, the 4K was rated better for brightness, contrast, and sharpness. **Conclusion:** Observer performance for detecting breast cancer on a 4K tablet PC with a high-resolution display is similar to that using a 5-MP LCD. This appears adequate for displaying mammograms of diagnostic quality and could be useful for patient consultations, clinical demonstrations, or educational and teaching purposes.

Keywords: breast cancer, mammography, soft-copy, tablet PC, 4K

1. Introduction

Since the introduction of the Apple iPad in April 2010, the use of the mobile tablet PC has increased rapidly and such devices now comprise a major portion of the PC market.

With new developments in technology, opportunities for the use of tablet PCs in hospitals for management or diagnosis have increased because of the great advantages they have in terms of portability and applications for teleradiology [1–4]. An increasing number of reports have compared the use of mobile device screens with liquid-crystal displays (LCDs) for diagnosis, and the accuracy of the former is now considered to be almost equal to that of the latter, or at least acceptable, for MRI diagnosis of spinal injury, radiography and CT diagnosis of intracranial hemorrhage and orthopedic injury, and CT diagnosis of pulmonary embolism [5–8].

The viewing of digital mammograms using a soft-copy reading device has many advantages in terms of image display, better handling, postprocessing capability, computer-assisted diagnosis, archiving of image information, and image data transmission [9]. High-grade (so-called medical purpose) LCDs, such as the 5-megapixel (MP) LCD, are recommended for soft-copy reading in digital mammography [10–12].

Recently, a high-resolution 4K color display has also been developed and is commercially available. 4K resolution refers to a display device or content having a horizontal resolution in the order of 4000 pixels. Several examples of 4K resolution exist in the fields of digital television and digital cinematography. To our knowledge, however, there is no definite consensus as to whether a 4K high-resolution display monitor would be acceptable for reading of mammograms. In terms of access, portability and cost effectiveness, it would be useful to clarify whether 4K images actually afford better diagnostic accuracy.

The purpose of this study was to assess the observer performance of 4K tablet PCs with a high-resolution calibrated grayscale display monitor for detection of breast cancers on digital mammograms, in comparison with 5-MP LCDs.

2. Methods and materials

2.1. Mammogram selection

The study cohort included 40 cases surgically verified and pathologically proven breast cancers (mean age, 51.2 years; age range, 29–83 years). Histologic analysis demonstrated invasive ductal carcinoma in 25 cases, ductal carcinoma *in situ* in 10, and special type in 5. The median size of the lesions revealed by pathologic examination was 18.3 mm (range 3–45 mm). In addition, 60 cases (mean age, 48.4 years; age range, 28–82 years) including 48 with normal breast findings and 12 with benign conditions (mastopathy in 6; cyst in 3; fibroadenoma in 2; papilloma in 1) were selected. Mention this in abstract as well. Finally, 100 cases (48 normal, 40 with cancer, and 12 with benign lesions) were examined. ACR BI-RADS for density, a predetermined breast density distribution was followed when selecting the cases: 10 were for cases with extremely dense breasts, 55 with heterogeneously dense breasts, 30 with scattered fibroglandular tissue, and 5 with entirely fatty breasts.

2.2. Image acquisition and display

Mammograms were acquired using a flat-panel digital mammography system (Senographe DS LaVerite; GE Healthcare). The spatial resolution was 100 μm per pixel (pixel dimension: 1800 × 2304) and the contrast resolution was 14 bits.

The images were displayed on two types of display: (i) two monochrome 5-MP LCDs (MFGD5621HD, 2048 × 2560 pixels, 21.3 inch; BARCO); and (ii) two commercially available 4K tablet PCs with high-resolution color monitors (4K UT-MA6, 2560 × 3840 pixels, 20.8 inch; Panasonic) (**Figures 1** and **2**).

The physical properties of the two types of monitors are shown in **Table 1**.

The displays run with the PACS software (We VIEW Z; HITACHI) and viewing software specialized for MGs (Plissimo MG, Panasonic). The luminance of both monitors was calibrated as recommended by the suppliers and at the start of the reading test.

2.3. Image interpretation

Four board-certified radiologists assessed the mammograms in a dark environment (<10 lux). Each of the observers independently assessed 200 images (100 patients × 2 sides; MLO and CC views). The observers were asked to rate the images on the level of confidence using the BI-RADS lexicon: 1, negative; 2, benign; 3, probably benign; 4, suspicious; and 5, highly suggestive of malignancy.

In addition, on another occasion, the observers assessed the image quality in terms of brightness, contrast, sharpness, and noise, side-by-side for the 5-MP LCDs versus the 4K tablet PCs (5-step Likert scale, −2 = 5-MP definitely better and +2 = 4K definitely better).

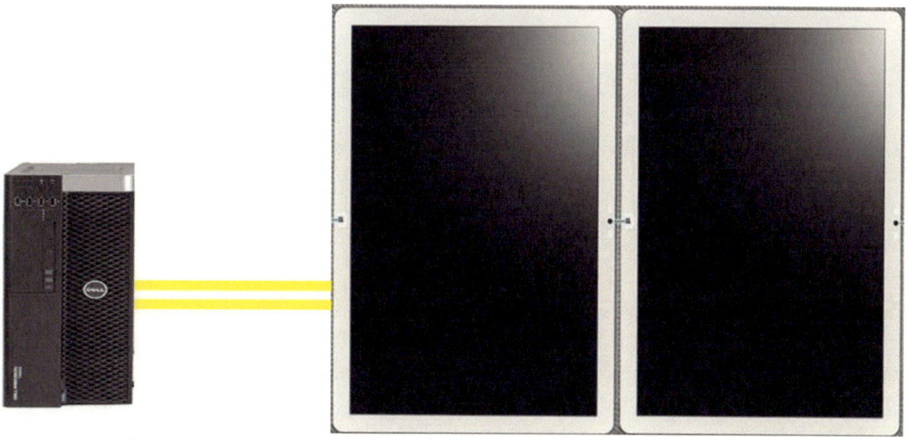

Figure 1. 4k UT-MA6 (TOUGHPAD) 20.8 inches; Panasonic.

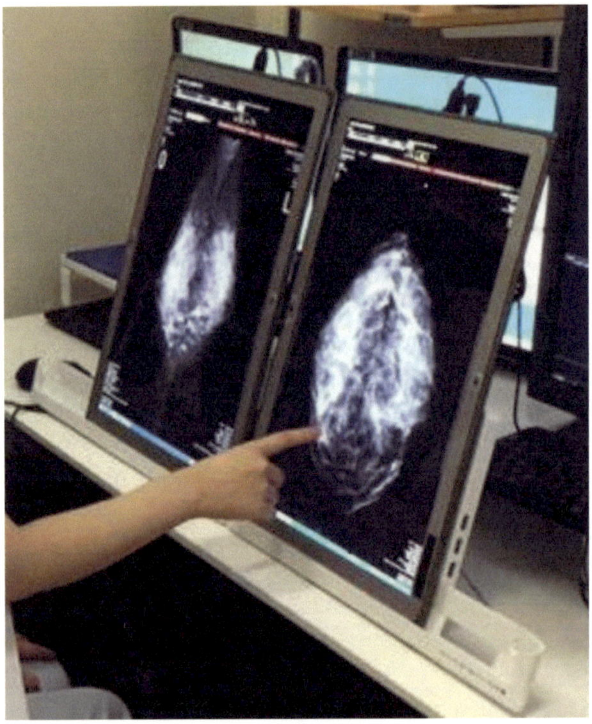

Figure 2. Two sets of 4K tablet PCs with high-resolution color monitors (4K UT-MA6, 2560 × 3840 pixels, 20.8 inch; Panasonic).

	Screen size	Matrix size	Color	Maximum luminance (cd/m²)	Contrast ratio	Product name (manufacturer)
4K tablet PC	20.8 (inches)	2560 × 3840	Color	300	850:1	UT-MA6 (Panasonic)
5-MP LCD	21.3 (inches)	2048 × 2560	Monochrome	450	800:1	MFGD5621HD (Barco)

Table 1. The physical properties of the 5-MP LCDs and 4K display monitors used in comparison with observer performance.

2.4. Data and statistical analysis

The observers' detection performance was evaluated using receiver operating characteristic (ROC) curve analysis. The confidence level results were used to construct ROC curves. This allowed to obtain the sensitivity, specificity, positive predictive value (PPV), negative predictive value (NPV), and accuracy of each monitor. Image quality ratings were tabulated for each reader and summarized across all readers. The confidence interval (CI) for the proportion of 4K ratings as similar (0), slightly better (±1), or better (±2) was obtained, considering the side-by-side comparison to be a single test condition. In the statistical analysis, differences at $P < 0.05$ were considered to be statistically significant.

3. Results

Table 2 and **Figure 3** show the average under the curve (AUC) values and ROC curves for detection of breast cancers using the 5-MP LCDs and the 4K tablet PCs, respectively. The mean AUC values for use of the 5-MP LCDs and the 4K tablet PCs were 0.921 and 0.936, respectively. The difference was not statistically significant ($P = 0.27$). Sensitivity, specificity, positive and negative predictive values, and accuracy were comparable (**Table 3**).

	BI-LADS	
	5-MP LCD	**4K**
Reader 1	0.858	0.903
Reader 2	0.932	0.954
Reader 3	0.945	0.945
Reader 4	0.949	0.958
Mean	0.921	0.936

Table 2. The area under the ROC curve for the 5-MP and 4K in BI-RADS scores.

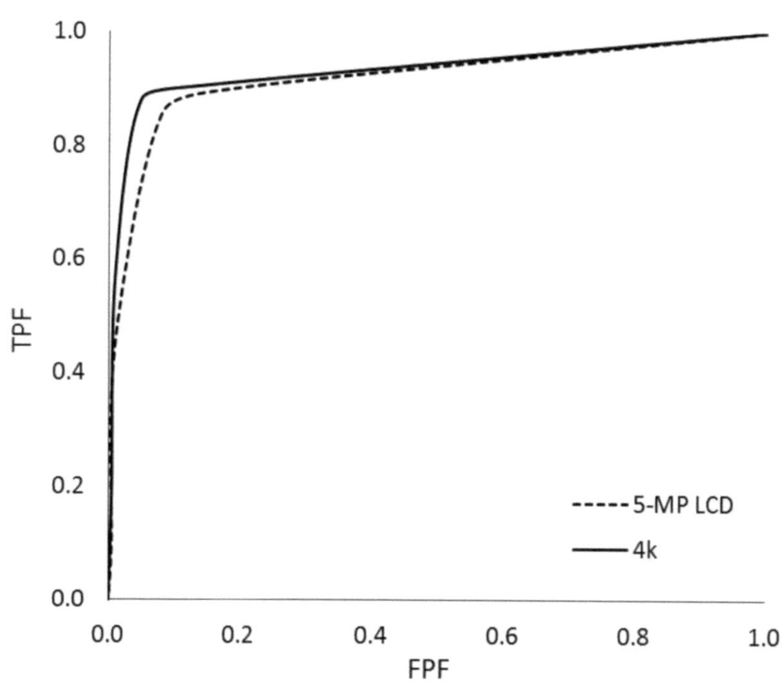

Figure 3. ROC curves for the detection of breast cancers. FPF, false positive fraction; TPF, true positive fraction. The thick line shows the ROC curve for a set of 4K tablet PC with high-resolution color monitors and the dashed line shows the ROC curve for a set of 5-MP LCDs. There was no significant difference between the two types of display modes ($P = 0.27$).

	5-MP LCD	4K
Sensitivity	0.857 (0.863/0.956)	0.881 (0.788/0.937)
Specificity	0.918 (0.889/0.936)	0.963 (0.939/0.978)
PPV	0.735 (0.643/0.794)	0.860 (0.769/0.915)
NPV	0.960 (0.931/0.980)	0.969 (0.945/0.984)
Accuracy	0.905 (0.860/0.934)	0.946 (0.908/0.969)

Table 3. Sensitivity, specificity, positive and negative predictive values and accuracy with the 5-MP and 4K.

With regard to image quality, brightness for the 4K tablet PC was rated as similar to that of the 5-MP LCD in 12% of the study readings, slightly better in 54%, and better in 27%. Contrast for the 4K tablet PC was rated as similar to that of the 5-MP LCD in 26% of the study readings, slightly better in 40%, and better in 15%. Sharpness for the 4K tablet PC was rated as similar to that of the 5-MP LCD in 38% of the study readings, slightly better in 26%, and better in 12%. Noise for the 4K tablet PC was rated as similar to that of the 5-MP LCD in 85% of the study readings, and slightly better in 5% (**Table 4** and **Figure 4**). **Figures 5–8** demonstrated breast cancers displayed on 5-MP and 4K monitors.

	4K better (+2)	4K slightly better (+1)	Similar (0)	5-MP slightly better (−1)	5-MP better (−2)	Mean	Lower 95% CL	Upper 95% CL
Brightness	27	54	12	7	0	1.00	0.84	1.16
Contrast	15	40	26	19	0	0.51	0.32	0.70
Sharpness	12	26	38	24	0	0.26	0.07	0.45
Noise	0	5	85	10	0	−0.05	−0.13	0.03

Table 4. Image quality on the basis of brightness, contrast, sharpness and noise, for side-by-side feature visibility rating with 5-MP versus 4K. Values are presented as numbers (also percentages). Mean is average preference by percentage. Positive numbers indicate a preference for 4K and negative numbers indicate a preference for 5-MP. CL; confidence limits.

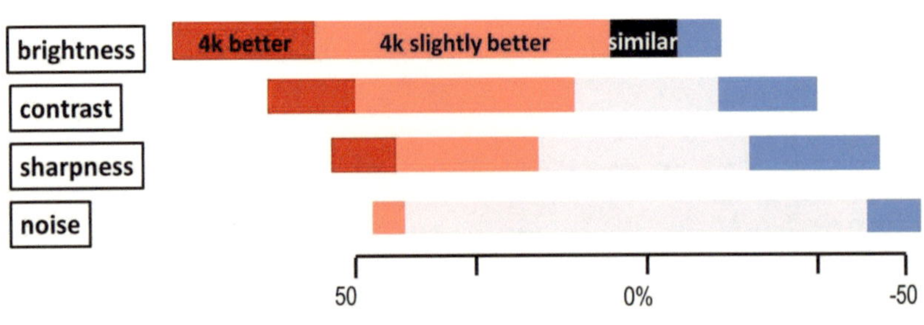

Figure 4. Likert scale scores (n = 100 eligible patients). Image quality on the basis of brightness, contrast, sharpness, and noise, for side-by-side feature visibility rating with 4K and 5-MP LCD. Values are presented as percentages.

http://dx.doi.org/10.5772/intechopen.69074

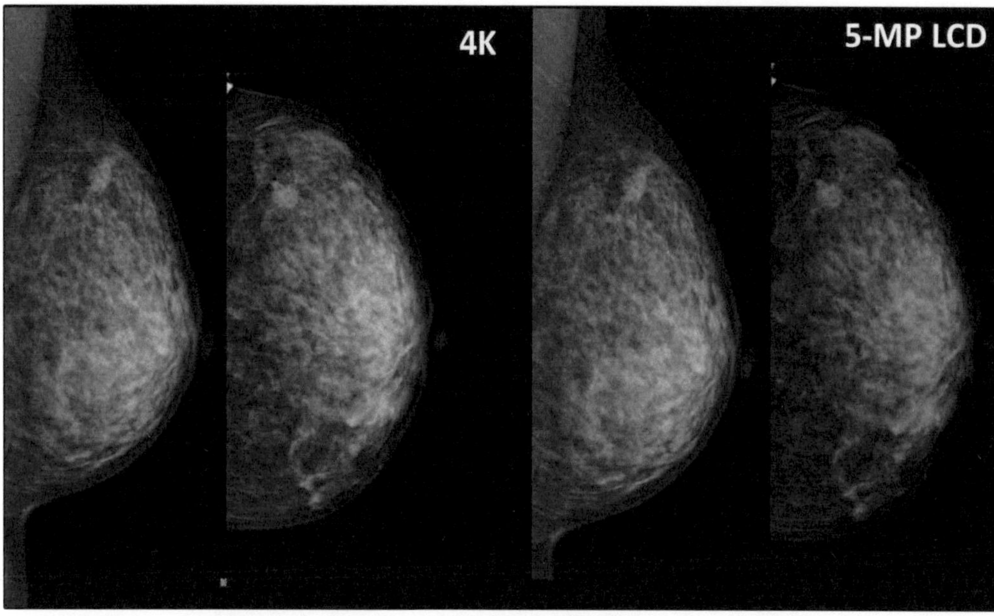

Figure 5. Microlobulated mass in the left upper area *captured images.

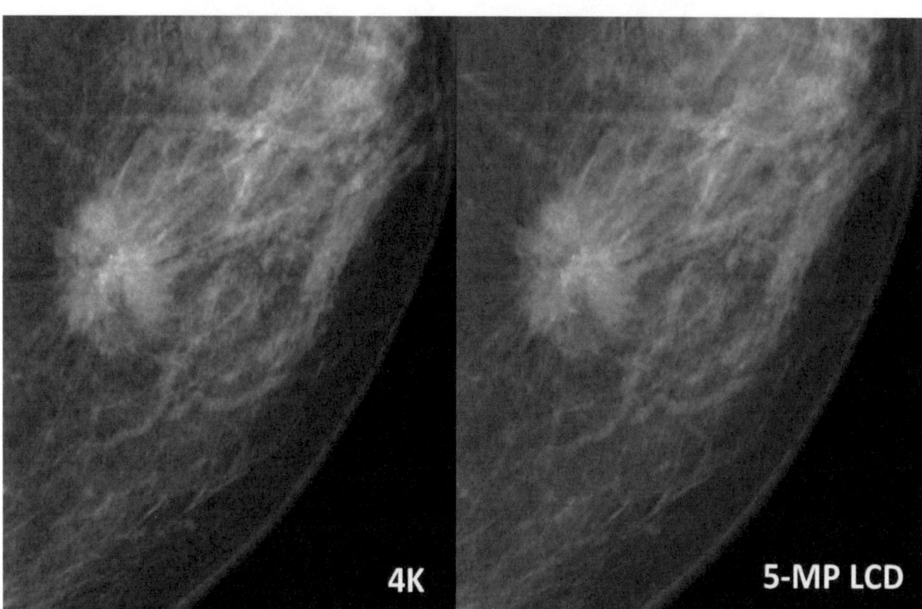

Figure 6. Spiculated mass *captured images.

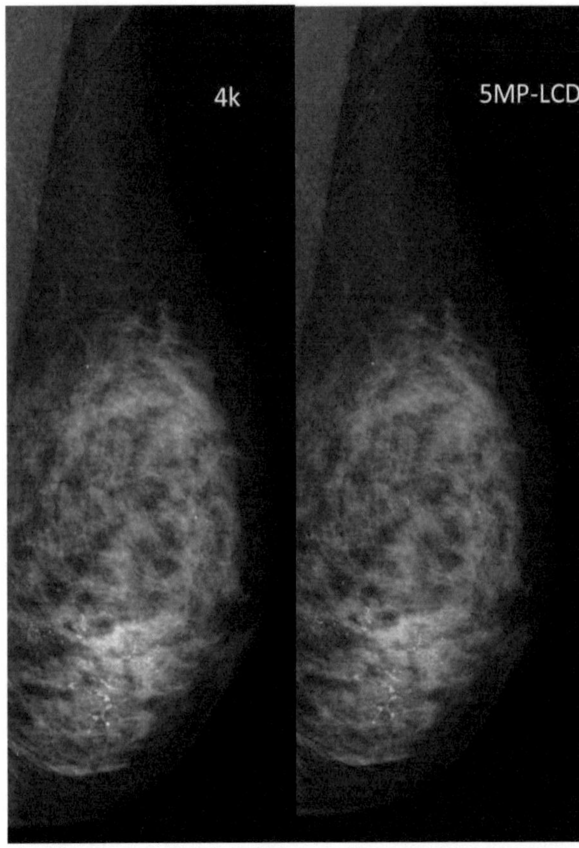

Figure 7. Finelinear branching calcifications in the left lower area *captured images.

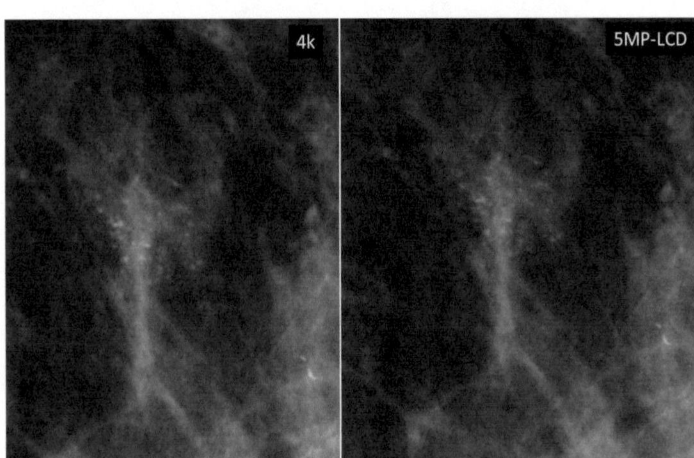

Figure 8. Amorphous grouped calcifications *captured images.

http://dx.doi.org/10.5772/intechopen.69074

4. Discussion

The purpose of the present study using images from actual patients was to obtain initial data to indicate whether or not the newer tablet PCs with a 4K high-resolution color display monitor could be deployed for mammographic imaging. Only one previous study has evaluated the display quality of tablet PCs [13]. This study represented the first attempt to evaluate the display quality of tablet PCs (iPad 2 and 3) with a dedicated 10-MP LCD using a standardized CDMAM phantom. It was concluded that the evaluated iPads, especially version 3, would likely be adequate for display of diagnostic-quality mammograms [13].

Our present study found no significant difference between the performances of the 5-MP LCDs and the 4K tablet PCs for detecting breast cancers on mammograms. Moreover, in terms of the image quality, 4K tablet PCs were rated as having better brightness, contrast, and sharpness. This is the first confirmation that observer performance for detection of breast cancers using soft-copy readings on digital mammograms is comparable between the current standard 5-MP LCDs and 4K tablet PCs with a high-resolution display monitor. The 4K tablet PC seems suitable for displaying mammograms in a variety of tasks such as patient consultation, clinical demonstrations, or educational and teaching purposes, and its large high-resolution screen seems to meet the legal requirements. As many patients are interested in taking a look at their images, one of the most promising applications of tablet PC-based mammographic display would be patient consultation. This would give patients a clearer idea of their disease and might have a positive impact on patient compliance.

The greatest benefits of the 4K tablet PC with a high-resolution display monitor are its low cost and possible application for multiple purposes, such as reporting systems and referencing of color images including endoscopic, PET/CT, and SPECT/CT images. In addition, the performance of 4K high-resolution color display monitors has recently improved, and they now have high-resolution (5-MP or more) capability, as is the case for medical LCDs. However, the development of tablet PCs is progressing rapidly; the 4K display used in the present study might now be considered a relatively old model. If the 4K display is suitable for medical display purposes, the cost would increase.

5. Conclusion

Our findings suggest that observer performance for detection of breast cancers on digital mammograms using 4K tablet PCs with a high-resolution display monitor is comparable to that obtained using 5-MP LCDs. Therefore, 4K tablet PCs, as a result of the advanced technology, might be adequate for diagnostic-quality mammogram display and could be useful for patient consultation, clinical demonstration, or educational and teaching purposes. Because of the promising potential advantages of tablet PCs, such as their portability, further assessments of their potential clinical use are warranted.

Author details

Ryusuke Murakami[1]*, Nachiko Uchiyama[2], Hitomi Tani[1] and Shinichiro Kumita[1]

*Address all correspondence to: rywakana@nms.ac.jp

1 Department of Radiology, Nippon Medical School, Tokyo, Japan

2 Department of Radiology, National Cancer Center, Tokyo, Japan

References

[1] Volonté F, Robert JH, Ratib O, Triponez F. A lung segmentectomy performed with 3D reconstruction images available on the operating table with an iPad. Interactive CardioVascular and Thoracic Surgery. 2011;**12**:1066-1068

[2] Mc Laughlin P, Neill SO, Fanning N, Mc Garrigle AM, Connor OJ, Wyse G, Maher MM. Emergency CT brain: Preliminary interpretation with a tablet device—Image quality and diagnostic performance of the Apple iPad. Emergency Radiology. 2012;**19**:127-133

[3] Takao H, Murayama Y, Ishibashi T, Karagiozov KL, Abe T. A new support system using a mobile device (smartphone) for diagnostic image display and treatment of stroke. Stroke. 2012;**43**:236-239

[4] Yoshimura K, Nihashi T, Ikeda M, Ando Y, Kawai H, Kawakami K, Kimura R, Okada Y, Okochi Y, Ota N, Tsuchiya K, Naganawa S. Comparison of liquid crystal display monitors calibrated with gray-scale standard display function and with γ 2.2 and iPad: Observer performance in detection of cerebral infarction on brain CT. American Journal of Roentgenology. 2013;**200**:1304-1309

[5] John S, Poh AC, Lim TC, Chan EH, Chong LR. The iPad tablet computer for mobile on-call radiology diagnosis? Auditing discrepancy in CT and MRI reporting. Journal of Digital Imaging. 2012;**25**:628-634

[6] McNulty JP, Ryan JT, Evanoff MG, Rainford LA. Flexible image evaluation: iPad versus secondary-class monitors for review of MR spinal emergency cases—A comparative study. Academic Radiology. 2012;**19**:1023-1028

[7] Toomey RJ, Ryan JT, McEntee MF, Evanoff MG, Chakraborty DP, McNulty JP, Manning DJ, Thomas EM, Brennan PC. Diagnostic efficacy of handheld devices for emergency radiology consultation. American Journal of Roentgenology. 2010;**194**:469-474

[8] Johnson PT1, Zimmerman SL, Heath D, Eng J, Horton KM, Scott WW, Fishman EK. The iPad as a mobile device for CT display and interpretation: Diagnostic accuracy for identification of pulmonary embolism. Emergency Radiology. 2012;**19**:323-327

[9] Kamitani T, Yabuuchi H, Matsuo Y, Setoguchi T, Sakai S, Okafuji T, Sunami S, Hatakenaka M, Ishii N, Kubo M, Tokunaga E, Yamamoto H, Honda H. Diagnostic performance in

differentiation of breast lesion on digital mammograms: Comparison among hard-copy film, 3-megapixel LCD monitor, and 5-megapixel LCD monitor. Clinical Imaging. 2011;**35**:341-345

[10] Yamada T, Suzuki A, Uchiyama N, Ohuchi N, Takahashi S. Diagnostic performance of detecting breast cancer on computed radiology (CR) mammograms: Comparison of hard copy film, 3-megapixel liquid-crystal-display (LCD) monitor and 5-megapixel LCD monitor. European Radiology. 2008;**18**:2363-2369

[11] Schueller G, Schueller-Weidekamm C, Pinker K, Memarsadeghi M, Weber M, Helbich TH. Comparison of 5-megapixel cathode ray tube monitors and 5-megapixel liquid crystal monitors for soft-copy reading in full-field digital mammography. European Journal of Radiology. 2010;**76**:68-72

[12] Yabuuchi H, Kawanami S, Kamitani T, Matsumura T, Yamasaki Y, Morishita J, Honda H. Detectability of BI-RADS category 3 or higher breast lesions and reading time on mammography: Comparison between 5-MP and 8-MP LCD monitors. Acta Radiologica. 2017;**58**:403-407

[13] Hammon M, Schlechtweg PM, Schulz-Wendtland R, Uder M, Schwab SA. iPads in breast imaging—A phantom study. Geburtshilfe Frauenheilkd. 2014;**74**:152-156

Chapter 8

Diagnostic System in Electrical Impedance Mammography: Background

Alexander Karpov, Andrey Kolobanov and
Marina Korotkova

Additional information is available at the end of the chapter

http://dx.doi.org/10.5772/intechopen.69195

Abstract

Electrical impedance mammography (EIM) belongs to nonlocal techniques of image creation. It is based on a number of data collection methods, including the cross-sectional approach, the back-projection method with the weight function applied horizontally and vertically, and the static image method. The analysis of data acquired by applying the above methods enabled to work out the EIM diagnostic system. It involves the following diagnostic categories: structural percentile limits and the mammary gland structure, age-related percentile limits and age-related electric conductivity, outlying values statistics and early diagnostics of breast cancer, D-statistics and distortion of the mammographic scheme in the presence of breast cancer, diagnostic table, and the assessment of the electrical impedance image.

Keywords: electroimpedance mammography, breast cancer, high-risk group

1. Introduction

Modern academic research and clinical practice avail of various tomography systems of electrical impedance diagnostics [1–7]. Electrical impedance mammography (EIM) represents one of the most rapidly developing imaging modalities designed for breast cancer detection [8–22].

EIM belongs to noninvasive techniques of image creation. It measures electromagnetic phenomena and assesses their changes via external scanning.

Since electric current distribution is not limited by two-dimensional plane, the data obtained reflect the change of electric conductivity in three-dimensional space, thus providing for the layer-by-layer image of the object. Based on the reconstruction of internal distribution from a set of external points, EIM refers to tomography techniques of image construction.

There exist two types of techniques creating tomographic images: local and nonlocal. The local technique implies the passage of one direct ray through the body causing the creation of one pixel in the image. The pixel value depends solely on the substance that the ray meets on its way. X-ray, magnetic resonance, and positron emission all belong to local or hard-field tomography techniques.

The nonlocal technique is characterized by all points on the object affecting the measurement result. This is the so-called cross measurement. The pixel value depends both on the object structure and the structure of the surrounding tissues. Electrical impedance, ultrasound reflection, and optical tomography belong to the category of nonlocal or soft-field tomography techniques.

Thus, EIM is a noninvasive technique featuring nonlocal properties of tomographic image creation.

2. Diagnostics system in electrical impedance mammography

Modern electrical impedance mammography systems, both commercial and experimental, differ in the following characteristics: alternating current parameters, electrode number and arrangement configuration, method of data collection, and algorithm of image reconstruction. Electrical impedance mammograph, MEIKv5.6, developed and manufactured by "PKF "Simtechnika," Russia was used for the creation of electrical impedance images [22].

The mammograph has the following significant characteristics:

- Noninvasive technology of image creation
- 3D-tomography system
- Form of "soft-field" tomography
- "Nonlocal" method of tomographic image creation
- 50 kHz frequency and 0.5 mA amplitude alternating current
- Planar positioning of electrodes
- 256 electrode panel
- Cross-sectional approach to data collection. The cross-sectional approach is a variation of the complementary method, when all electrodes are involved in measurement pairwise.
- Back-projection method as an algorithm of image reconstruction
- Static image
- Quantitative diagnostic information

The analysis of data obtained via the MEIKv5.6 electrical impedance mammograph allowed to pick out the following diagnostic categories:

- Structural percentile limits and mammary gland structure
- Age-related percentile limits and age-related electric conductivity
- Outlier statistics and early detection of breast cancer
- D-statistics and distorted mammographic scheme in the presence of breast cancer
- Diagnostic table and EIM image evaluation

2.1. Structural percentile limits and mammary gland structure

The analysis in hand is based on data acquired from 1632 electromammographic examinations of normal women of various age groups. It is essential that the test groups contained about the same number of women: 380 women aged 20–30, 428 women aged 31–40, 449 women aged 41–50, and 375 women aged 51–60. The analysis of the electrical impedance mammograms was carried out "blindly", i.e., without taking the women's age into account.

The fluctuations of the electrical impedance index values made from 0.01 standard units, the lower range value, to 0.68 standard units, the upper range value. To define the structure of electric conductivity index distribution, we extracted eight property ranges with the 0.09 step and calculated the number of observations in each range (**Table 1**).

Figure 1 shows data distribution by the electric conductivity index. The conductivity index mean value constituted 0.29, median, and 0.26, mode.

A bell-shaped curve, similar mean, median, and mode values allow us to declare the quantitative variable (electric conductivity index in this case) distribution as normal. Mean value and

Electric conductivity index	Number of observations
0.05–0.14	0
0.15–0.24	67
0.25–0.34	279
0.35–0.44	471
0.45–0.54	435
055–0.64	299
0.65–0.74	75
0.75–0.84	6
Total	1632

Table 1. Distribution of mean electric conductivity index frequencies.

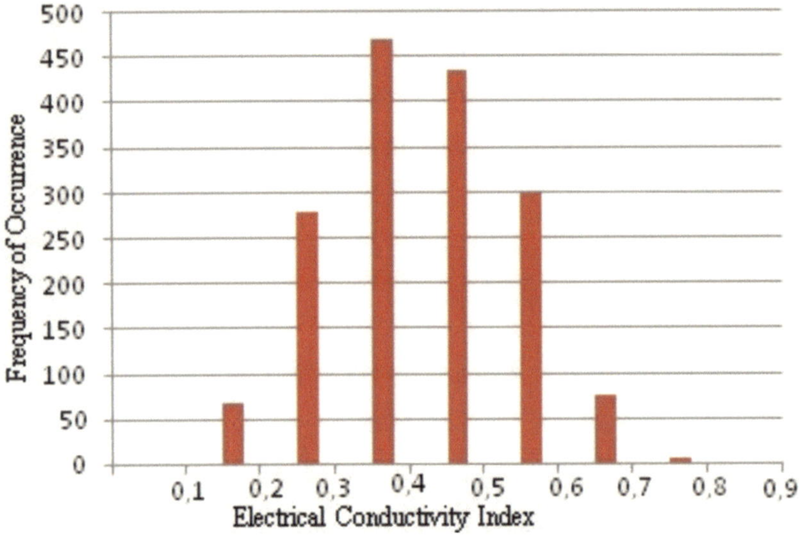

Figure 1. Histogram of mean electric conductivity index frequency distribution.

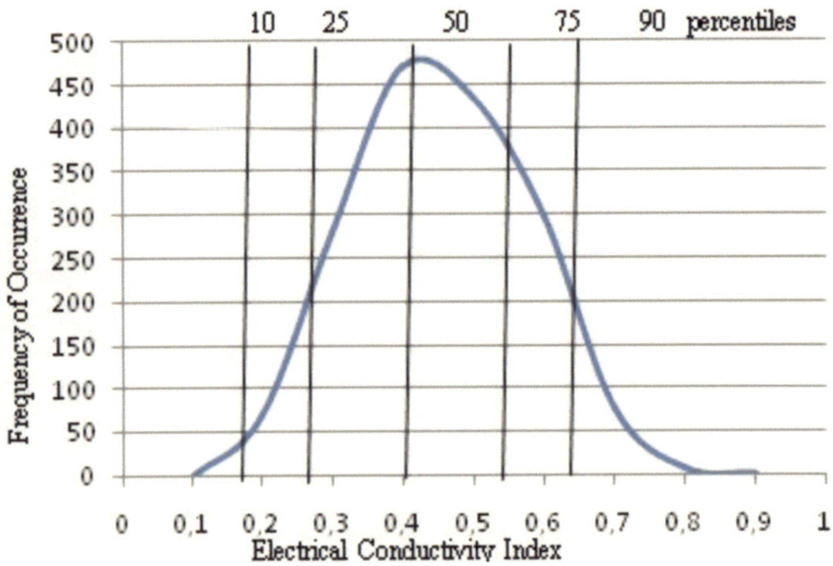

Figure 2. Frequency polygon and percentile ranges.

standard deviation are generally used for normal distribution characterization. We see the implementation of the 10th, 25th, 50th, 75th, and 90th percentile as most rational since it does not require the knowledge of the variable distribution form (**Figure 2**).

In accordance with the proposed assessments, the values within the first range (below the 10th percentile) should be considered as distinctly low, within the second range (10th–25th percentile) as low, the third and fourth ranges (25th–75th percentile) as mean, within the fifth range (75th–90th percentile) as high, and the sixth range (above the 90th percentile) as distinctly high.

The mammary gland structure allows to distinguish a few kinds of tissues performing various functions (epithelial, connective, nerve, blood, and lymph). The age involution of the mammary gland consists in the reduction of ductal epithelium proliferation, in the substitution of the secretory epithelium by a connective tissue with different correlations of tissue elements. The electric conductivity index (IC) obtained from the electrical impedance scanning is a quantitative variable, which characterizes the mammary gland structure. A low index is typical of a gland containing a big number of cell elements and thereafter high ion concentration. This causes us to regard the mammary gland structure with the conductivity index percentile limit <10 percentile as representing the ductal type. This is confirmed by the fact that the proportion of the test-group women aged 20–30 with the ductal type of the mammary gland structure and indices fitting in the first channel (<10 percentile) exceeded 70%. A high electric conductivity index is typical of a gland containing big number of fat lobules and a lot of connective tissue and therefore low ion concentration. Thus, the mammary gland structure with the conductivity index percentile limit >90 percentile should be estimated as representing the amorphous type. This is confirmed by the fact that the proportion of women aged 51–60 with the involutive type of the mammary gland structure and indices fitting in the sixth channel (>90 percentile) also exceeded 70%. The mammary gland structure with the conductivity index percentile limit between the 25th and 75th percentile should be estimated as representing the mixed type. This is proved by the fact that this percentile channel included data of women of all age-groups. Different combinations of structures determining tissue electric conductivity produce a wide range of conductivity index values.

Table 2 presents a summary table of the mammary gland structure assessment from the perspective of EIM execution.

Thus, the mammary gland structure can be assessed from the perspective of electrical impedance mammography with a view to the electric conductivity index. As is well-known, the mammary gland structure conditions its density, which is why the distinguished ranges of electric conductivity correspond to different types of breast density. The so-called dense breasts, which correlate with the ductal structural type, are characterized by low values of

Structural type	Electric conductivity	Percentile limits
Amorphous	Above 0.66	>90‰
Mixed with the predominance of the amorphous component	0.57–0.65	75–90‰
Mixed	0.30–0.56	25–75‰
Mixed with the predominance of the ductal component	0.22–0.29	10–25‰
Ductal	Below 0.22	<10‰

Table 2. Types of mammary gland structure from the perspective of electrical impedance mammography.

electric conductivity index. High index values are typical of the amorphous structure when the mammary gland chiefly consists of the adipose and connective tissues. The peculiarity of this approach to the mammary gland structure assessment is a quantitative expression of the mamma's anatomic and histological composition. The results of the mammary gland density assessment from the perspective of electrical impedance mammography with a view to the electric conductivity index are presented in **Table 3**. The assessment is done in line with the American College of Radiology (ACR) terms [23].

2.2. Age-related percentile limits and age-related electric conductivity

The analysis in hand is based on data acquired from over 2000 electromammographic examinations of normal women aged 20–80. The analysis of the electrical impedance mammograms was carried out using the percentile limits approach, the women's age taken into account. It should be noted that modern medical, biological, and clinical research has been increasingly employing the percentile approach as a method of concise description of distributions. This approach does not require the knowledge of distribution form, i.e., it is nonparametric. The use of percentile curves is routine for many diagnostic modalities, e.g., they are widely used for the assessment of fetal development in ultrasound diagnostics. 5, 50, and 95 percentile limits for the electric conductivity index were calculated in each age group, which allowed to draw percentile curves (**Figure 3**) and make a table summarizing percentile limits of normal age-related electric conductivity of the mammary glands (**Table 4**).

Percentile limits of age-related electric conductivity can be used for the formation of breast cancer risk groups. The conductivity index values below the 5th percentile must be regarded as distinctly low, whereas the values exceeding the 95th percentile as distinctly high.

The risk group for breast cancer should thus include patients exhibiting abnormally low age-related electric conductivity values, i.e., below the 5th percentile, which witnesses for extremely high density of the glandular tissue ductal component. High density of the ductal

	EIM classification	**Electric conductivity**	*ACR classification*
Type Ia	Amorphous	above 0.66	Predominantly fat, parenchyma below 25%
Type Ib	Mixed with the predominance of the amorphous component	0.57–0.65	
Type II	Mixed	0.30–0.56	Fat with some fibroglandular tissue, parenchyma between 25 and 50%
Type III	Mixed with the predominance of the ductal component, high density of the ductal component	0.22–0.29	Heterogeneously dense, parenchyma 50–75%
Type IV	Ductal, extremely high density of the ductal component	below 0.22	Extremely dense, parenchyma 75–100%

Table 3. Mammary gland structure and density types from the perspective of EIM execution in accordance with the ACR classification.

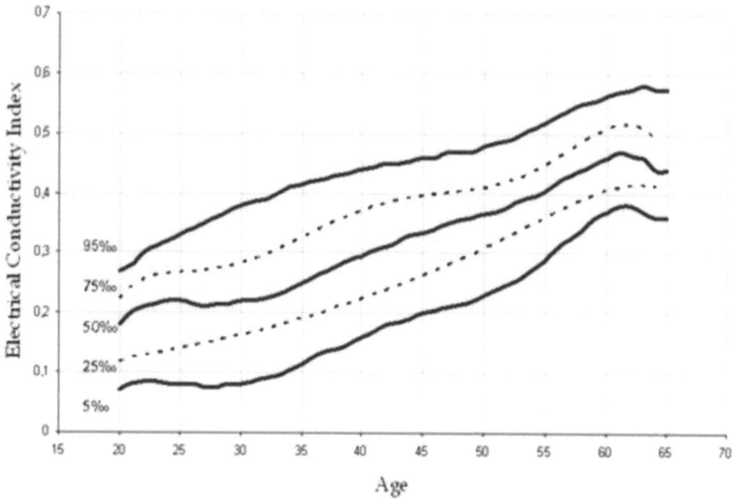

Figure 3. Percentile curves of age-related electric conductivity of the mammary gland.

Age range, years	5 percentile	50 percentile	95 percentile
20–29	0.18	0.28	0.44
30–39	0.16	0.40	0.53
40–49	0.22	0.51	0.63
50–59	0.32	0.58	0.72
60–69	0.43	0.57	0.78
over 70	0.50	0.57	0.64

Table 4. Age-related percentile limits of the mean electric conductivity index.

component carries potential threat since it is often conjoined by the insufficient trophic function of the connective tissue, which is known to be provided by the main substance thereof. Dyscrasia may result in dystrophic processes, including those in the basal membrane.

Abnormally high values of age-related electric conductivity, i.e., exceeding the 95th percentile, correlate with menstrual disorders, the latter standing for hormonal changes.

2.3. Outlier statistics and early detection of breast cancer

Unlike other tomographic modalities which only avail of visual evaluation feature, electrical impedance scanning also provides quantitative information. These unique data are used for diagnostic purposes. A detailed description thereof demands a short reference to outlier statistics.

Provided that all value variations come from a single general population, they are expected to differentiate by virtue of random causes only and stay within the range of M ± 2 standard deviation. However, we sometimes come across values, which differ dramatically from the rest of the totality. Such values are often referred to as outliers. In this case, checking the values for the presence of outliers is highly desirable. If such a difference is a result of an error or its cause is unknown, the outlier value should be excluded from the assessment. Elimination of values that are "too remote" from the center of a sample is called sample *censoring*.

There are two basic types of methods implemented for outlier elimination [24]:

(a) Elimination method with the general standard deviation given.

(b) Elimination method with the general standard square deviation not given.

In the first case, *X* and standard deviation are calculated with a view to the results obtained from the sample aggregate; in the second case, the sample is stripped of the suspicious results before the calculations are made. Normalized deviate, which serves a nondimensional characteristic of the variable deviation from the arithmetical mean, is one of the criteria used to determine the outliers (1).

$$t = x - M/\sigma \tag{1}$$

where "t" is the outlier detection criterion, "x" is an outlier, "M" is the mean value for a variant group, and "σ" is a standard deviation. "ttable" stands for standard values of the outlier detection criterion, the values are shown in the table. The values of ttable= 2, P = 0.95 are often used for large selections.

The "three sigma" rule applied for the assessment of the measurement results distributed in accordance with the normal law is one of the simplest outlier detection methods. This rule implies the following: if $Xoutlier - X > 3S_x$, where S_x–is an assessment of the standard deviation measurement, the result is hardly probable and may be considered as a miss. The *X* and S_x values are calculated without regard to the extreme values of *Xoutlier*.

In this paragraph, we will comment on the results of an electrochemical test of the MEIK v5.6 electrical impedance mammograph. The figure below shows a prototype installation filled with water. The mammograph was used to acquire an electrical impedance scan of the physiological saline solution (**Figure 4A**). The mean electric conductivity index (IC) made 1.85,

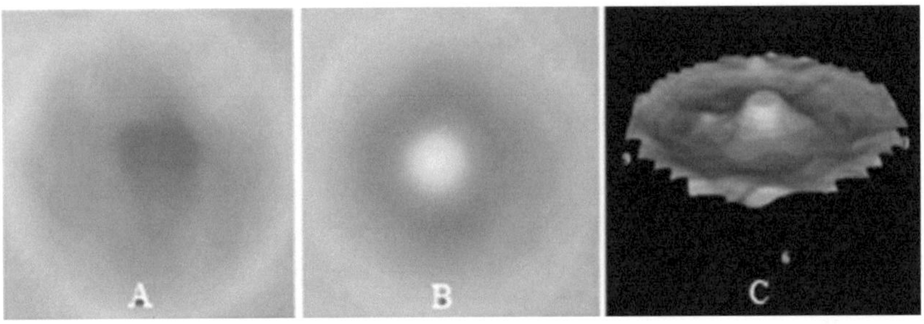

Figure 4. Electroimpedance scans (11 mm deep) of water: A–homogeneous, B–with a metal coin in the middle, C–a 3D image.

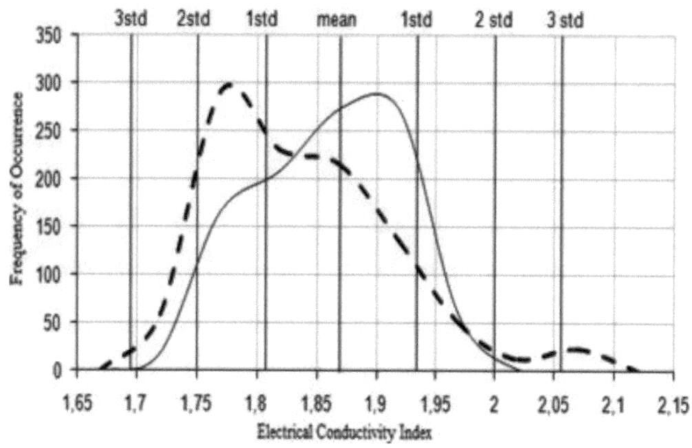

Figure 5. Histograms of electric conductivity distribution of water (continuous curve) and of water with a coin (dotted curve).

whereas the standard deviation amounted to 0.075 and three standard deviations to 0.22. Then, a metal coin was put into the water, 1 cm deeper than the mammograph panel with electrodes (**Figure 4B**). When overlapped, the conductivity distribution histograms (**Figure 5**) allow to see that the IC of the coin (dotted curve) is higher than the IC of water (continuous curve) by a value exceeding three standard deviations. This is typical of outliers; however, in this particular case, it speaks for the presence of an object whose IC value is significantly different from that of the medium, neither does the object belong to the general observation population.

The above mentioned fully applies to medical and biological measurements. **Figure 6** shows an electrical impedance mammogram of a patient suffering from breast cancer, the quantitative parameters being: IC = 0.56, standard deviation–0.12. At 3 o'clock next to the areola, we can see an indistinctly contoured focus with the IC of 0.94. Thus, the IC in the area of interest exceeds the IC of the mammogram by a value going over 3 standard deviations. On the right, we present X-ray and ultrasound images of the same case.

The given example proves that the electric properties of malignant tumors differ significantly from those of the surrounding tissue. It is a well-known fact that cancer cells exhibit an increased electrical activity. Some of the characteristic features of cancer cells that affect their electrical activity are:

1. Cancer cells have cell membranes that exhibit different electrochemical properties and a different distribution of electrical charges than normal tissues [25].
2. A change in mineral content of the cell, particularly an increase in the intracellular concentration of positively charged sodium ions and an increase in the negative charges on the cell coat (glycocalyx) are two of the major factors causing cancer cells to have lower membrane potential than normal cells [25].
3. Cancer cells exhibit both lower electrical membrane potentials and lower electrical impedance than normal cells [26, 27].

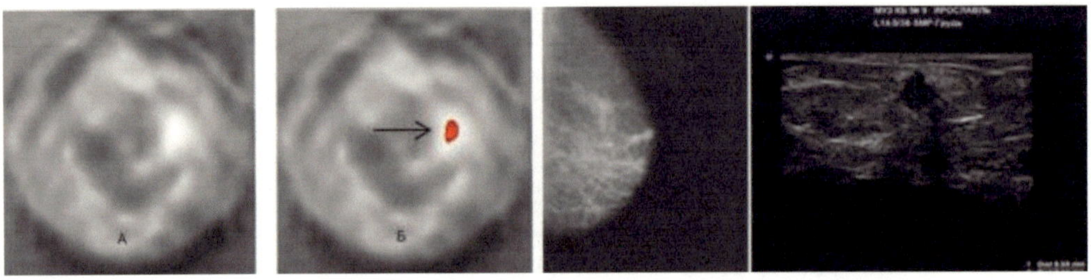

Figure 6. On 3 o'clock next to the areola, a focus is visualized (A), highlighted–arrow (B), less than 10 mm in size. X-ray: A lesion of less than 1 cm in size with a radiant contour in the upper-outer segment. US: a lesion of an irregular shape, with nonhomogeneous structure, 9 × 9 mm without vascularization.

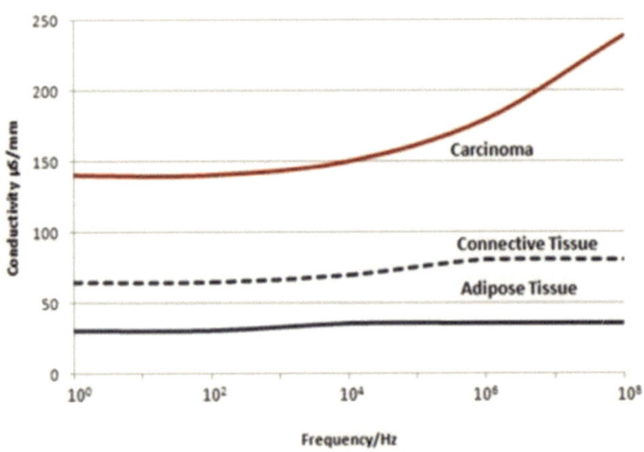

Figure 7. Influence of the current frequency on the electric conductivity of the mammary gland tissues.

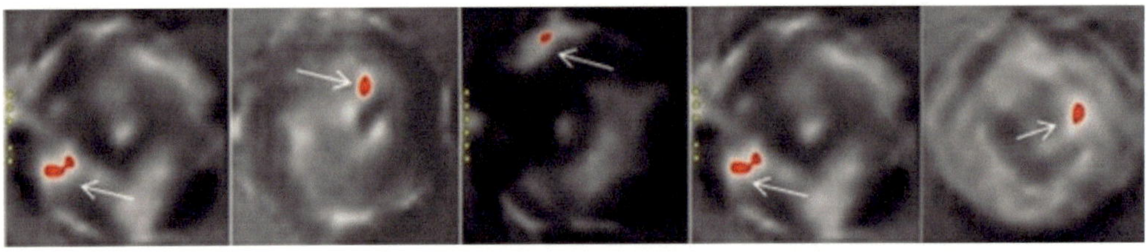

Figure 8. High electrical conductivity area (>3 std) outside the lactiferous sinus zone, which is highlighted (arrow).

From **Figure 7**, it becomes clear that the mammary gland carcinoma has three times higher electric conductivity than the surrounding tissues [28].

This knowledge can be applied to early detection of breast cancer. To perform this task one is to search for areas with abnormal values of IC>3 std, which is typical of an oncologic process with tumors not exceeding 1 cm. To make the search easier, the mammograph highlights abnormal conductivity areas with red (arrow) (**Figure 8**).

2.4. D-statistics and distorted mammographic scheme in the presence of breast cancer

As the disease connected by the breakup of the epithelium basal membrane progresses, various phenomena can occur in the tumor and the surrounding tissues. These processes are always accompanied by alterations of electrical properties of the tumor mass. Increased vascularization leads to electrical conductivity increase due to ionic conduction. Replacement of dead tumor cells by collagen fibers leads to electrical conductivity decrease. While purulent inflammation areas emerge, permittivity decreases as a result of the cell membranes death. Lymphocytic infiltration causes the tumor and the surrounding tissues impedance to increase, because of a significant local concentration of cell membranes. Thus, tumor growth is regularly accompanied by the alteration of the electrical properties both of the tumor and the surrounding tissues.

As noted previously, the electrical impedance approach enables to conduct a quantitative analysis of the image involving the assessment of the following parameters: mean electric conductivity index, histogram of electric conductivity distribution, comparison of the electric conductivity distribution histogram with the referent values.

To refer the patient to the norm or pathology category, the divergence in the distribution form criterion, also known as the λ-criterion or the Kolmogorov-Smirnov criterion [29], is used in Eq. (2).

$$\lambda = \left|\sum N1(xij)/n1 - \sum N2(xij)/n2\right| \max\sqrt{n1n2/n1+n2} \tag{2}$$

where *N1* stands for observation quantities within the ranges, *n1*–within the sample aggregate, A_1; and *N2* and *n2*–the same for A_2.

Dx statistics, to be more exact, a subaggregate when calculating the Kolmogorov-Smirnov criterion Eq. (3).

$$D(xij) = \left|\sum N1(xij)/n1 - \sum N2(xij)/n2\right| \max \tag{3}$$

where *N1* stands for observation quantities within the ranges, *n1*–within the sample aggregate, A_1; *N2* and *n2*–the same for A_2.

This nonparametric criterion enables to determine the statistical significance of divergences in the distribution of any characteristic of norm or pathology including the distribution of electric conductivity on electrical impedance tomograms.

The Dx statistics allows to define the area of one of the distributions, which is not shared by the other (**Figure 9**). The Dx value reflects the proportion of observations or data, which distinguishes experiment (patient) from control (norm). This value is essential for substantiation of diagnosis as well as for assessing the parameter information capacity.

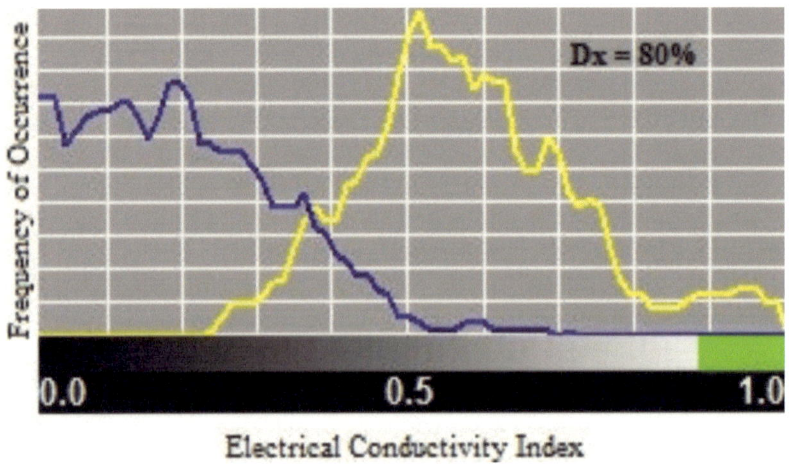

Figure 9. Assessment of distribution divergence by their area.

High information capacity of the divergences revealed enables to refer the patient to this or that category (e.g., norm or cancer) with great probability. To determine the informative value of distribution divergence Kulback's information measure is applied Eq. (4).

$$J = 10\,\lg P1/P2 * 0.5(P1 - P2) \tag{4}$$

where J = information value of the range, $P1$–probability of patients' suffering from disease A1 getting into the range, $P2$–the same for disease A2.

It shows how informative the Dx statistics applied is, how this parameter contributes to diagnosing the disease, e.g., cancer. The assessment of distribution divergence (Dx) produced results standing in direct relationship with the information capacity, according to Kulback (**Table 5**). This relationship must be recognized as fairly regular and consistent [29].

In the presence of cancer, the histogram of the affected gland is shifted. **Table 6** sums up data on comparative electric conductivity obtained from patients suffering breast cancer, benign changes of the mammary gland as well as from normal women with different types of mammary gland structure.

In the course of oncologic process development, general and local electric conductivity naturally tends to change. The distortion of the mammographic scheme can be observed as early

Distribution divergence	Information capacity	Reliability
below 20%	Very low	No
20–30%	Relatively low	Yes
30–50%	Good	Yes
50–65%	High	Yes

Table 5. Distribution divergence and information capacity.

	Number of patients	Comparative electric conductivity (affected–normal gland)					
		<20%	20–30%	30–40%	40–50%	50–60%	>60%
Cancer	310	101 (33%)	67 (22%)	44 (14%)	37 (12%)	26 (8%)	35 (11%)
Healthy	161	157 (98%)	4 (2%)	0	0	0	0
Healthy acinar-ductal type	20	18 (90%)	1 (5%)	1 (5%)	0	0	0
Healthy amorphous type	32	28 (88%)	2 (6%)	2 (6%)	0	0	0
Benign	68	59 (87%)	7 (10%)	2 (3%)	0	0	0

Table 6. Comparative electric conductivity of the mammary glands, data acquired from patients suffering from breast cancer, benign lesions, and normal women.

Diagnostic criteria	Electrical impedance mammography points
Shape	
• Round, oval	1
• Lobular, irregular	2
Contour	
• No	0
• Sharp	1
• Hyperimpedance, indistinct	2
Surrounding tissues	
• *Preserved*	0
• Structure alteration/displacement	1
• Thickening/extrusion/retraction	2
Internal electrical structure	
• Hyperimpedance ($IC_{roi} < IC_{av} - 2std$)	0
• Isoimpedance$IC_{roi} = IC_{av} \pm 2std$)	1
• Hypoimpedance ($IC_{roi} > IC_{av} + 2std$)	2
• Animpedance ($IC_{roi} > IC_{av} + 3std$)	3
Comparative electrical conductivity	
• Divergence between the histograms <20%	0
• Divergence between the histograms 20–30%	1
• Divergence between the histograms 30–40%	2
• Divergence between the histograms >40%	3

Table 7. Diagnostic criteria for differentiation of volumetric lesions in electroimpedance mammography.

as at onset of the disease that is why this criterion was added to the EIM breast cancer diagnostic scale (**Table 7**). Below (**Figure 10**), we provide examples of the distorted mammographic scheme from three patients with breast cancer.

2.5. Diagnostic table and EIM image assessment

A volumetric lesion is an extensional involvement detected on several scan planes. Image analysis implies the assessment of the lesion shape, contour, internal electric structure, and changes in the surrounding tissues.

A diagnostic table was made to regularize the description of volumetric lesions. **Table 7** presents assessment parameters each being given a certain set of points.

Using the numerical score for the assessment of volumetric lesions in electrical impedance mammography allows to compare this information to BI-RADS ACR categories (**Table 8**).

The EIM point scale enables to standardize the description of volumetric lesions when carrying out electrical impedance mammography examination as well as use the algorithm of patients' supervision worked out by the specialists of the American College of Radiology.

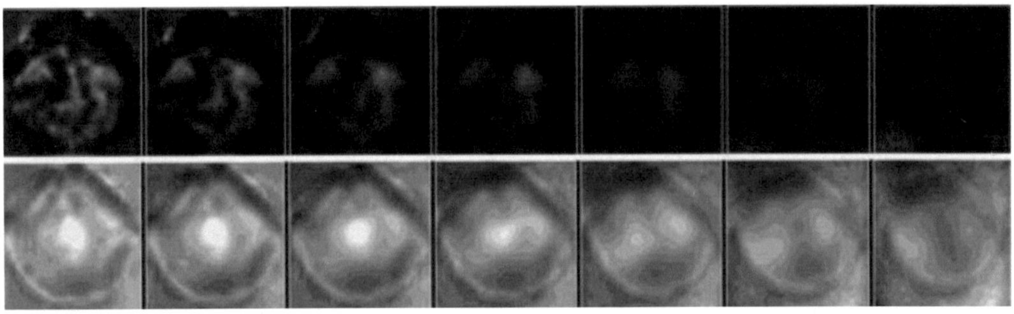

Figure 10. Electroimpedance mammographic scheme distortion (the top images show the affected gland, the bottom line contains images of the normal breast).

EIM	**ACR**
Common scale	*BI-RADS categories*
No score	BI-RADS 0 poor image
0–1	BI-RADS 1 lesion is not defined
2–3	BI-RADS 2 benign tumors–routine mammography
4	BI-RADS 3 probably benign findings
5–7	BI-RADS 4 suspicious abnormality–biopsy
>8	BI-RADS 5 highly suggestive of malignancy–treatment/biopsy

Table 8. EIM scale and ACR BI-RADS.

3. Conclusion

EIM diagnostic system is a clear and logical system involving determination of the mammary gland structure and density, allowing for cancer diagnostics for various types of breast as well as formation of breast cancer risk groups.

Author details

Alexander Karpov*, Andrey Kolobanov and Marina Korotkova

*Address all correspondence to: karpovay@medyar.ru

Clinical Hospital, Yaroslavl, Russia

References

[1] Barber DC, Brown BH. Applied potential tomography. Journal of Physics E-Scientific Instruments. 1984;**17**(9):723-733

[2] Brown BH, Seagar AD. The Sheffield data collection system. Clinical Physics and Physiological Measurement. 1987;**8**(Suppl A):91-97

[3] Electrical impedance tomography. Edited by D.S.Holder, IOP. 2005

[4] Karpov A, Korotkova M, et al. Electrical impedance potential mammography for visualization of objects (Electrochemical tests). Journal of Physics: Conference Series. 2010;**224**:012032

[5] Akhtari-Zavare M, Latiff L. Electrical impedance tomography as a primary screening technique for breast cancer detection. Asian Pacific Journal of Cancer Prevention. 2015;**16**(14):5595-5597

[6] Shetiye P, Ghatol A, et al. Detection of breast cancer using electrical impedance and RBF neural network. International Journal of Information and Electronics Engineering. 2015;**5**(5):P356-360

[7] Prasad NS, Houserkova D, Campbell J. Breast imaging using 3D electrical impedance tomography. Biomedical Papers of the Medical Faculty of the University of Palacky, Olomouc Czechoslovakia. 2008;**152**(1):151-154

[8] Cherepenin V, Karpov A, Korjenevsky A, Kornienko V, Mazaletskaya A, Mazurov D, Meister D. A 3D electrical impedance tomography (EIT) system for breast cancer detection. Physiological Measurement. 2001;**22**:9-18

[9] Cherepenin V, Karpov A, Korjenevsky A, Kornienko V, Kultiasov Y., Ochapkin M,Trochanova O, Meister J. Three-dimensional EIT imaging of breast tissues: System design and clinical testing. Medical Imaging. 2002;**V21**N6:662-667

[10] Karpov A, Korjenevsky A, Mazurov D, Mazaletskaya A. 3D electrical impedance scanning of breast cancer. World Congress on Medical Physics and Biomedical Engineering, Chicago; 2000; p. 62

[11] Halter RJ, Hartov A, Paulsen KD. A broadband high-frequency electrical impedance tomography system for breast imaging. IEEE Transactions on Biomedical Engineering. 2008;**55**(2 Pt 1):650-659

[12] Jossinet J. A hardware design for imaging the electrical impedance of the breast. Clinical Physics and Physiological Measurement. 1988;**9**Suppl A:25-28

[13] Kerner TE, Paulsen KD, Hartov A, Soho SK, Poplack SP. Electrical impedance spectroscopy of the breast: Clinical imaging results in 26 subjects. IEEE Transactions on Medical Imaging. 2002;**21**(6):77-80, 95-100

[14] Kim, BS, Boverman, G, Newell, JC, Saulnier, GJ, Isaacson, D. The complete electrode model for EIT in a mammography geometry. Physiological Measurement. 2007;**28**(7):S57-S69

[15] Raneta O., Ondruš D., Bella V. Utilisation of electrical impedance tomography in breast cancer diagnosis. Klinická Onkologie. 2012;**25**(1):36-41

[16] Karpov A, Korotkova M. Diagnostic criteria for mass lesions differentiating in electrical impedance mammography. Journal of Physics: Conference Series. 2013;**434**:012053

[17] Chakraborti K, Selvamurthy W. Clinical application of electrical impedance tomography in the present health scenario of India. Journal of Physics: Conference Series. 2010;**224**:012069

[18] Zain N., Kanaga K. A review on breast electrical impedance tomography clinical accuracy. ARPN Journal of Engineering and Applied Sciences. v2015;**10(**15):P6230-6234

[19] Pak D, Rozkova N, et al. The electroimpedance computer tomography in screening of diseases of the breast. Medical Visualization. 2012;**2**:P35-42

[20] Zain N, Chelliah K. Breast imaging using electrical impedance tomography: Correlation of quantitative assessment with visual interpretation. Asian Pacific Journal of Cancer Prevention. 2014;**15**(3):1327-1331

[21] Korotkova M, Karpov A, et al. Electrical impedance imaging characteristics of nodular and edematous-infiltrative forms of breast cancer. Breast Cancer Symposium. San Antonio. 2011:6-10

[22] Korotkova M, Karpov A. Standards for Electrical Impedance Mammography In book "Imaging of the Breast. Technical Aspects and Clinical Implication". Edited by Tabar L, Croatia, 2014

[23] Breast Imaging Reporting and Data System (BI-RADS). 4th ed. Reston: American College of Radiology; 2003

[24] Zaydel A. Error of Measurement of Physical Quantities. 1985

[25] Cure JC. On the electrical characteristics of cancer. Paper presented at the Second International Congress of Electrochemical Treatment of Cancer. 1995; Florida

[26] Cone CD. Variation of the transmembrane potential level as a basic mechanism of mitosis control. Oncology. 1970;**24**:438-470

[27] Blad B, Baldetorp B. Impedance spectra of tumour tissue in comparison with normal tissue: A possible clinical application for electrical impedance tomography. Physiological Measurement. 1996;**17**Suppl 4A:A105-A115

[28] Jossinet J. The impedivity of freshly excised human breast tissue. Physiological Measurement. 1998;**19**:61-75

[29] Gubler E. Quantitative methods for analysis and identification of pathology. Leningrad. 1978

Chapter 9

An Innovative Concept of 3D X-Ray Imaging Systems for Painless Breast Cancer Detection

Mohammed Ali Alnafea

Additional information is available at the end of the chapter

http://dx.doi.org/10.5772/intechopen.70385

Abstract

Breast cancer is a life-threatening disease and considered one of the most common forms of cancer among women worldwide. Early and accurate detection with mass screening programmes helps improve a woman's chances for successful treatment. The current and the most effective technique used for screening and diagnosis of breast cancer is the X-ray mammography. The photon transport detection of such technique is mostly based on a forward scattering mechanism as well as makes use of attenuation and penetration coefficients. The painful compression and the double X-ray exposure of both patients' breasts carried out during the imaging process remain unavoidable. In addition, the conventional 2D mammography has two major limitations: sensitivity in detecting breast cancers (~ <80%) and the high recall rate (~10%). It suffers from certain limitations, most important of which is tissue overlap and false diagnoses arising thereof. To overcome this and as an alternative, a new 3D imaging method for breast cancer screening and diagnosis, namely, tomosynthesis, has recently been used. In such method, a limited number of low-dose 2D projection images of a patient are used to reconstruct the 3D tissue information. Tomosynthesis systems incorporate an X-ray source that moves over a certain angle to acquire images. This tube motion is a major limitation because it degrades image quality, increases the scan time and causes prolonged patient discomfort. Therefore, the goal of this work was to overcome all of the above limitations by developing an innovative proof of concept for painless 3D X-ray mammography to be hopefully used as a screening and as diagnostic methods for breast cancer detection by utilizing the scattered X-ray photon information. Most imaging modalities required a wide spectrum of capabilities, which span biomedical sciences, physical sciences and clinical medicine; thus, the ongoing methodology aims to establish a collaborative cross-disciplinary research engaging together with scientists in universities and clinicians in hospitals. Consequently, we hope that this work provides the potential to score some successes in clinical imaging science. In order to do this and since it is generally not possible or feasible to use real components to build and optimize a system repeatedly, a Monte Carlo simulation was used. The first phase focused on realistic computer simulation of the proposed imaging system to find the optimum setup as well as to aid in the analysis of the effect of various factors on the system performance. Thus, the main focus was on 3D mammography imaging simulation setup. Five main steps have been carefully checked and successfully produced: (a) the production of X-ray radiation or source after careful and detailed physics check. This includes the interaction between the X-ray photons and the object (the 3D breast phantom) that is used on scan as well as the detector system and its associated electronics modelled. (b) Next is the realistic modelling of anthropomorphic breast phantoms to check if the effectiveness of prediction of the simulation is successfully achieved. A computer simulation model is developed to estimate the radiation dose to the breast that would be incurred using mammography. Mono-energetic normalized glandular dose coefficients, DgN(E), were computed for energies 11–120 keV using breast phantoms of various sizes and compositions.

Keywords: mammography, breast cancer detection, 3D imaging

1. Introduction

Breast cancer is one of the most common cancers in Saudi Arabia [1] and, thus, is an important health problem [2]. In the Western world, it is the second most frequent cause of cancer death in women (after lung cancer) [3]. Statistics show that a large number of women in Europe, North America, Australia and many Latin-American countries suffer from this life-threatening disease [4]. Worldwide, in the year 2005, the number of new cases exceeded 1.2 million [3]. Breast cancer is rare in women below the age of 20 years and less common below the age of 30 years, but it is more aggressive and thus has a lower survival rate. The incidence rate, however, rises dramatically over the age of 50 years. This could be due to several risk factors such as family history, genetics, early menstruation, late menopause and other factors that have not yet been identified. Breast cancer can also occur in males and often fatal, but it is extremely rare. The above problems have prompted global governments to put constant efforts to increase patient's recovery level against this disease. Early and accurate detection with mass screening programmes helps improve a woman's chances for successful treatment. It also minimizes pain, suffering and anxiety that surround patients and their families.

The current and the most cost-effective technique used for screening and diagnosis of breast cancer is X-ray mammography. It is the state of the art for earlier detection to improve both prognosis and survival rate [5]. This may be due to its good availability, high sensitivity and relatively low cost/patient. Despite the above efforts, the mortality rate of breast cancer still remains high and in the UK, for example, accounts for ~17% of all female deaths [6, 7]. This is due to some limitations of the current mammographic procedures. As a result, a large number of cases with positive mammography results undergo invasive surgical breast biopsies. Breast biopsy is still widely used and thus is the only fail-safe method to determine whether a lesion is malignant. Of all biopsy cases, only about 25% prove to be malignant. Moreover, a majority of the diagnosed women below the age of 50 have a dense breast tissue. This is a problem as it obscures lesions and results in false-negative mammography.

In addition, the size, shape and appearance of the female breast are not constant but undergo a number of changes during the lifetime of women. For instance, changes occur during the menstrual cycle and more pre-/postmenopause. In addition, the age of the subject not only influences the shape but also parenchymal density of the breast. Thus younger women tend to have denser breasts (more fibro-glandular tissue), whilst postmenopausal women have breasts containing a larger adipose component. This makes the X-ray mammogram far more effective in older women as the fat content is more radio-translucent (appears darker) than glandular tissue (appears underexposed) in younger women [8].

The above discussion suggests that both the shape and parenchymal density of the breast impose particular constraints on the choice of imaging modality. The imaging technique should be powerful for initial detection and subsequent follow-up of the diseases. At present, no single technique can be used for all cases of breast cancer detection without showing certain clinical or technical limitations. This implies necessity to address the specific needs that can help for breast tumour imaging to overcome these limitations. For instance, breast compression is often needed as it holds the breast still and enhances the spatial resolution. It also evens out the breast thickness and reduces scatter in X-ray or gamma-ray imaging in case of scintimammography (SM) [9], thus increasing image sharpness. Moreover, it spreads out the tissue so that small abnormalities will not be obscured by the overlying breast tissue. Since the breast is an external organ and extends to the chest wall, it requires appropriate views to be taken. For instance, in X-ray mammography a lateral (from the side) view of the breast allows separation of the chest wall from lesions deep within the breast.

Furthermore, mammography involves the radiological examination of the breast using equipment specifically designed for, and dedicated to, imaging breast tissue. This equipment is primarily used for the detection of breast cancer at an early stage. It is widely used in screening programme involving healthy populations of women. Early detection of breast cancer in a healthy population places particular demands on radiological equipment as high-quality images are required at a low dose. Symptomatic patients may also benefit from the development of mammography equipment that produces high-quality images for breast screening. Perhaps because of the exacting demands of mammography, acceptability criteria and suspension levels are well developed [10, 11]. It has been an accepted practice that mammography should be performed on X-ray equipment designed and dedicated specifically for imaging breast tissue, due to the clinical imaging requirements for high-quality image. In practice, either film/screen or digital detectors may be used. Both qualitative and quantitative acceptability criteria have been published for X-ray mammography by considering the image quality needed clinically in screening programmed.

2. Literature review

Cancer is a disease that starts in a localized organ or tissue and then grows out of control. Breast cancer is an important health problem as in the western world; it is the second most frequent cause of cancer death in women (after lung cancer) [6, 7]. Statistics show that a large number of women in Europe, North America, Australia and many Latin-American countries suffer from this life-threatening disease [8]. Worldwide, in the year 2005, the number of new cases exceeded 1.2 million [7]. Breast cancer is a heterogeneous disease as it has different cell types and different behavioural characteristics and appearances. Understanding the types of breast cancer and their growth pattern is important for imaging purposes. Breast cancer is usually categorized into two main types: invasive (infiltrating) and non-invasive (in situ) cancer. In situ means that the cancer cells are at early stage, i.e. remains localized to ducts (milk passages) or lobule (milk producing glands) with no micro-invasion to the surrounding fatty tissue. Once the basement membrane is penetrated, the cancer cells break into the surrounding tissue and are referred to as invasive breast carcinoma. Breast cancer is rare in women below the age of 20 years and less common below the age of 30 years, but it is more aggressive and thus has a lower survival rate. The incidence rate, however, rises dramatically over the age of 50 years. This is may be due to several risk factors such as family history, genetics, early menstruation, late menopause and other factors that have not yet been identified. Breast cancer can also occur in males and often fatal, but it is extremely rare. The above problems have prompted global governments to put constant efforts to increase patient's recovery level against this disease. Early and accurate detection with mass screening programmes helps improve a woman's chances for successful treatment. It also minimizes pain, suffering and anxiety that surround patients and their families. The current and the most cost-effective technique used for screening and diagnosis of breast cancer is X-ray mammography. It is the state of the art for earlier detection to improve both prognosis and survival rate [9].

Mammography is a low-energy (25–32 keV) X-ray examination of the soft tissues of the breast. It uses the variation in density between normal mammary features and abnormal tissue structures (lesion) to produce the image. The current widely used technique is based on screen-film technology. It is considered the gold standard in breast imaging as it is fast and available and has a lower cost than the scintimammography. It has two main applications: as a screening method in asymptomatic patients and as a diagnostic method in symptomatic populations. The former application is extremely important, and its introduction has significantly reduced the mortality rate of breast cancer in many countries [10, 11]. The American Cancer Society (ACS), the Department of Health and Human Services (HHS), the American Medical Association (AMA) and the American College of Radiology (ACR) recommend screening mammography every year for women, beginning at age 40. This is because the screening services accurately detect micro-calcifications and non-palpable soft tissue masses which until now have been beyond other imaging methods thanks to the high spatial resolution (50100 μm). Research has shown that annual mammograms lead to early detection of breast cancers, when they are most curable and breast-conservation therapies are available. The National Cancer Institute (NCI) adds that women who have had breast cancer and those who are at increased risk due to a genetic history of breast cancer should seek expert medical advice about whether they should begin screening before age 40 and about the frequency of screening. A recent review [12] estimated that screening leads to a reduction in breast cancer mortality of 15 and to 30% overdiagnosis and overtreatment. This means that for every 2000 women invited for screening throughout 10 years, one will have her life prolonged. In addition, 10 healthy women, who would not have been diagnosed if there had not been screening, will be diagnosed as breast cancer patients and will be treated unnecessarily. Furthermore, more than 200 women will experience important psychological distress for many months because of false-positive findings. Normally, screening is achieved by exposing the breast to X-rays after being gently compressed between two plates and then taking two views for each breast. A craniocaudal (imaging from above to below) and lateral views are generally taken. A lead grid is used to reduce scattering photons that reach the film. Diagnostic mammography is used for assessing the size of the lesion, for pre-surgical localization of suspicious areas of breast and in the guidance of needle biopsies.

The reported sensitivity (the fraction of patients actually having the disease and correctly diagnosed as positive) in lesion detection varies between 69 and 90% [13] depending on the breast density. The specificity (the fraction of patients without the disease, correctly diagnosed as negative) is the major drawbacks of conventional mammography. A variation in specificity between 87 and 97% and a low positive predictive value as low as 15% have also been reported in Ref. [14]. This 'less than perfect' performance may be due to several confounding factors, e.g. poor mammographic technique, observer error, the lesions are non-palpable or at a cellular level and/or the lesions are obscured by the normal breast tissues. In addition, the presence of scars or tissue distortion may hide true small tumours on the mammogram. Moreover, in mammography the ultimate challenge with regard to X-ray image quality and, thus, improving the reliability of screening and early diagnosis, requires better epidemiological understanding of breast tissues, improved diagnostic tools, enhanced quality control, continuous training and efficient management of data and records. Nevertheless, conventional mammography remains the most valuable and cost-effective technique for breast tumour diagnosis.

Over the last two decades, considerable efforts have been carried out to improve the current screen-film mammographic technique. These improvements include image quality, acquisition techniques and interpretation protocol in order to reduce some of the mammographic limitations [15]. Furthermore, a new research effort started 5 years ago focusing on 'digital mammography' (DM) as a possible future direction in breast imaging. Digital mammography, also called full-field digital mammography (FFDM), is a mammography system in which the X-ray film is replaced by solid-state detectors that convert X-rays into electrical signals. These detectors are similar to those found in digital cameras. The electrical signals are used to produce images of the breast that can be seen on a computer screen or printed on special film similar to conventional mammograms. This technique offers many advantages compared to the conventional screen-film-based method [16, 17]. For instance, processing with digital systems increases dynamic range (two to four times the dynamic range of typical film screen) and improved quantum efficiency and storage and display mechanisms. In addition, the use of computer-assisted image interpretation is claimed to be helpful for the physician. This may enhance different features such as computer-aided diagnosis which may further improve the visibility of lesions and improve mammographic sensitivity [18]. Therefore, repeated exposures (which are sometimes needed when using conventional mammography) are not required, and this may reduce the radiation dose. Moreover, it does not need either cassettes or dark rooms or processors and thus allegedly saves space and time in archiving and retrieving DM images. However, DM requires large disk space for saving image data.

Despite several advantages, DM does not yet replace screen-film mammography in many centres. However, with continuous technical improvements of the digital system, it is gradually taking over the conventional systems. Both conventional and DM systems suffer from substantial technical and clinical limitations. For instance, these systems are unreliable in imaging patients with dense parenchyma tissue especially in the younger female population due to more glandular tissue. Breast implants can also impede accurate mammogram readings because both silicone and saline implants are not transparent on X-rays. Thus, it blocks a clear view of the tissues behind them. This is true especially if the implant has been placed in front of, rather than beneath, the chest muscles. This issue requires an experienced technologists and radiologists to carefully compress the breasts to improve the view without rupturing the implant. All the above limitations and problems of imaging need to be dealt with to enhance detection efficiency and overcome the drawback. One of the methods that recently employed is the computer-aided detection (CAD) systems. Such systems use a digitized mammographic image that can be obtained from either a conventional film mammogram or a digitally acquired mammogram. The computer software then searches for abnormal areas of density, mass or calcification that may indicate the presence of cancer. The CAD system highlights these areas on the images, alerting the radiologist to the need for further analysis. Despite that mammographic findings are non-specific (cannot always differentiate benign from malignant disease) and often underestimate the size of the detected lesion, X-ray–based imaging is also not useful for breast diagnosis following surgery or radiotherapy as the patient's breasts in these cases have architectural distortion. Mammography is not recommended for women with breast implants and is also not useful following hormonal replacement therapy due to the increase of breast density. It is worth mentioning that X-ray mammography is not always useful for non-palpable tumours. Another group of women—close carrying a mutation in BRCA1 (human gene called breast cancer 1, early onset) or BRCA2 (breast cancer 2) genes—are at high genetic risk of cancer, some even having opted for preventative bilateral mastectomy. It is preferred not to repeat scan this group due to X-ray dose, and thus, a more sensitive diagnostic test would be advisable.

Moreover, the size, shape and appearance of the female breast are not constant but undergo a number of changes during the lifetime of women. For instance, changes occur with pregnancy, breast feeding and during the menstrual cycle. In addition, the age of the subject not only influences the shape but also parenchymal density of the breast. That is why young women tend to have dense breasts (more fibro-glandular tissue), creating a rounded appearance. On the other hand, postmenopausal women have breasts containing a large amount of fat. This makes the X-ray mammogram far more effective in older women as the fat content is more radio-translucent (appears darker) than glandular tissue (appears underexposed) in younger women [19]. The above discussion suggests that both the shape and parenchymal density of the breast imposes particular constraints on the choice of imaging modality. The imaging technique should be powerful for initial detection and subsequent follow-up of the diseases. At present, no single technique can be used for all cases of breast cancer detection without showing certain clinical or technical limitations. This implies necessity to address the specific needs that can help for breast tumour imaging to overcome these limitations. For instance, breast compression is often needed as it holds the breast still and enhances the spatial resolution. It also evens out the breast thickness and reduces scatter in X-ray or gamma-ray imaging [20], thus increasing image sharpness. Moreover, it spreads out the tissue so that small abnormalities will not be obscured by the overlying breast tissue. Since

http://dx.doi.org/10.5772/intechopen.70385

the breast is an external organ and extends to the chest wall, it requires appropriate views to be taken. For instance, in X-ray mammography a lateral (from the side) view of the breast allows separation of the chest wall from lesions deep within the breast. On the other hand, in single photon-ray emission imaging, one needs to separate the breast from the heart by employing an appropriate prone (face down) position. However, it has been claimed that with prone imaging view, there is a possibility of missing a small low-intensity medial lesion because of attenuation. This implies that another image is needed but with the camera positioned in the lateral view. In addition, shielding the camera from the background cardiac flux is very useful in tumour detection in terms of contrast and resolution [21, 22].

Having discussed the golden diagnostic technique for breast tumour imaging, the following section will describe the complementary imaging techniques of the breast. The image reconstruction techniques will be then discussed. Section 3 will be closed by presenting some preliminary results and a description of the design details.

3. Complementary diagnostic techniques

From the previous discussion, it is clear that there are some clinical situations where there are significant limitations to use mammography in isolation. In such cases, there is a great need to use sensitive tests to achieve a high confidence and accurate diagnostic decision. The use of breast biopsies is necessary if breast cancer is indicated or suspected in such cases. Of the performed breast biopsies, about 60–80% [23] are negative breast cancer or have benign lesions. In these cases, breast biopsies are considered unnecessary. This has led many breast cancer experts to propose complementary imaging modalities to provide additional diagnostic information and reduce unnecessary breast biopsies.

Ultrasonography (US) uses high-frequency acoustic waves that reflect at boundaries with different acoustic properties. It is a non-invasive technique, easily available and relatively cheap. Breast US provides unique information in assessing both palpable and non-palpable breast abnormalities. For instance, it clearly differentiates between solid masses and cystic lesions [24]. It is also considered to be useful in cancer staging, measuring tumour sizes, easy accessing lesions located in peripheries and reducing the number of unnecessary biopsies. It allows accurate needle placement during biopsy and is very useful for aspiration of cysts. The members of the European group for breast cancer screening recommended using US as a complementary method to X-ray mammography. In addition, the use of high-frequency transducers has improved spatial resolution and thus claimed to be useful in axillary node evaluation. However, breast US technique is time-consuming and operator/observer dependent. It has also a number of other limitations that may be due to overlapping in sonographic characteristics. For instance, it cannot detect calcifications (micro-calcifications or macro-calcifications) in DCIS. It could also miss solid lesions especially in a fatty breast and if detected cannot determine whether a solid lump is benign or malignant. For these reasons, US is not used as a screening technique for asymptomatic breast cancer as it is difficult to ensure that the entire breast has been scanned.

Magnetic resonance imaging (MRI) images are created by the recording of signals generated after radio-frequency excitation of nuclear particles exposed to strong magnetic field. Breast MRI is a non-ionizing tomographic functional technique that may be used when the diagnosis is uncertain with mammography [25]. The technique is valuable for specific clinical indications such as patients with (1) axillary adenopathy (enlargement or inflammation of the lymph gland), (2) possible tumour recurrence after surgery or radiotherapy, (3) lesions overlying implants or (4) those requiring staging of multifocal carcinoma (two or more discrete lesions in one breast) [26]. Breast MRI with dedicated breast coil has excellent soft tissue resolution that enhances the ability to both identify the location and in some cases determine the full extent of the lesion. The use of intravenous contrast agent, gadolinium, which accumulates in tissues with a dense blood vessel network, has also increased the sensitivity of breast MRI [13]. However, the reported specificity (ability to determine if lesion is benign or malignant) is 56–72% [27]. This technique has a limited application in patients with implanted metal devices or other metallic materials inside the body. MRI cannot also differentiate between inflammatory breast cancer and abscesses. In addition, several clinical limitations have been reported in the literature suggested not to use MRI in premenopausal women. For example, changes that do occur in the T1 value of the breast tissue during the menstrual cycle [13] mean that patients should be scanned between the 6th and 16th days of the cycle. In summary, researchers have concluded that breast MRI is limited by lack of availability and inconsistent quality, and the technique is too expensive for routine use in breast cancer screening.

The need to improve the breast cancer detection and to reduce the unnecessary invasive breast biopsies has stimulated researchers to investigate functional imaging modalities. These techniques produce a range of different imaging approaches such as positron emission tomography (PET), single-photon emission computed tomography (SPECT), planar imaging and dedicated imaging instrumentation with and without breast compression. These imaging techniques of the breast potentially over additional information in breast cancer diagnosis. This is because these imaging methods rely on the physiological and biochemical characteristics of a lesion. Thus, they are considered as the best hope to differentiate between benign/normal and malignant diseases. These functional techniques have also been used to assess and monitor the effect of cancer prevention drugs. The current radionuclide imaging techniques used for breast tumour imaging are briefly discussed.

In PET a small amount of positron emitter radio-tracer, 18fluorodeoxyglucose (FDG), is administered intravenously to the patient [27]. It is then distributed in the body, and as it decays, the radionuclide emits a positron in any random direction. If the positron whilst travelling interacts with an electron within the body, the two particles then annihilate and produce two rays of 511 keV each. Either a whole-body scanner or a breast-specific positron emission mammography (PEM) camera [28] is used to detect the two gamma-rays in coincidence (two events that are detected within ~ 12 ns). PEM is increasingly used in North America not only in cancer diagnosis but also in staging, planning and monitoring anticancer therapy. This information can be helpful not only in eliminating unnecessary axillary dissection [29] and biopsies but also in determining the appropriate treatment. The diagnosis of viable tumour tissue following chemotherapy is another application of PET [30, 31]. Imaging with 18F-FDG has shown considerable promise in breast cancer imaging, but the exact role is still in evolution. Wahl [32] recommended that it is best applied to solve difficult clinical cases in specific patients rather than routinely. There are a number of reasons that limit the wide use of PEM for routine cancer diagnosis: (1) the high cost (over $2 million) of PET coincidence imaging equipment, i.e. cyclotron, scanner and radiochemistry facility [27]; (2) the difficulty of producing and labelling the short half-life PET radionuclides [28]; (3) the lack of centres with the required experience to develop more advanced methodology appropriate for breast oncology—in particular, more data are needed about the metabolism of different PET radiopharmaceuticals in breast tumours—and (4) the lack of oncologists with a high knowledge of PET methodology [32].

Scintimammography (SM) is a promising non-invasive functional imaging technique. It has been proposed to complement X-ray mammography and to improve patient selection for biopsy. This single-photon imaging of the breast involves injecting the patient in the arm vein with a small amount (555–740 MBq [33]) of radiopharmaceutical. The most commonly used radiopharmaceutical for SM is ^{99m}Tc labelled Sestamibi. After a period of time, the tracer distributes in the breast tissue as well as in the body organs. It accumulates more in the target object (lesion) with uptake ratio nearly 9:1 tumour-to-background ratio (TBR) [43]. A standard full-size clinical gamma camera is then used to scan the patient and thus measure the 3D distribution of the radioactivity. SM imaging using full-size clinical camera includes a range of different imaging approaches such as planar (2D) imaging or SPECT technique. The latter technique gives a 3D representation image but is not widely used because it is difficult with this technique to accurately localize the lesion [40]. In contrast, planar SM is the technique that is more widely used in clinical practice because it provides better lesion localization particularly the prone images with lateral views [34]. In this case the gamma camera is usually equipped with a LEHR parallel-hole collimator, and two views (prone and supine) are taken to the diagnosed breast. Since the energy imaged is 140 keV representing the photo peak, 20% energy window (symmetric ~10%) is often used and thus centred over the photo peak.

In brief, SM with a general-purpose camera has been introduced to evaluate patients with dense breast prior and in a least case after breast biopsy [35]. The technique may also be considered valuable for many clinical applications such as evaluating the axillary lymph nodes, investigating patients with microcalcifications [36], assessing multifocal and multicentric breast cancer diseases [37]. It is also useful for imaging patients following surgery, chemotherapy, hormonal replacement therapy and radiotherapy as well as for patients with breast implants [34]. The technique may also assist in the differentiation of benign and malignant breast abnormalities by measuring radio-tracer uptake in the lesions as compared with surrounding breast tissues. Studies such as [38, 39] suggested that SM may be used as a second-line diagnostic test in cases where the sensitivity of mammography is decreased or there is doubt about the presence of lesion. In summary, SM using conventional camera may be considered as a useful complementary imaging modality to aid the diagnosis and the detection of breast cancer [40]. It may also help to assess in patient selection for biopsies, and this may reduce the number of unnecessary or negative breast biopsies. However, the major drawback of the current standard clinical gamma camera SM imaging systems is the use of mechanical collimator. This causes the camera imaging system to utilize a very small fraction, ~0.01%, of the total number of the emitted photons. This limits the statistics and hence the quality and diagnostic value of the observed images. The collimator sensitivity and resolution are a trade-off, and the camera is also limited by its intrinsic spatial resolution. As a result, these factors make it difficult to practically image cases of smaller, non-palpable, lesions (<1 cm) that may be deep seated or those close to the chest wall. These have stimulated the development of new dedicated (breast specific) instrumentations that are used for breast tumour imaging applications.

Recent years have seen considerable interest by scientists in developing new compact medical imaging detectors. These instruments were proposed for different clinical applications with the aim to improve image quality by building cameras of suitable size and shape for the part of the body under investigation. Among these designed detectors is the small dedicated gamma camera for functional breast tumour imaging. The justification for this development is that a standard full-size clinical gamma camera is designed for whole-body imaging and, thus, has not been optimized for breast tumour imaging. In other words, there are a number of shortcomings with such general-purpose gamma camera such as the limiting sensitivity (on average 50% [41]) for lesions <1 cm such as DCIS particularly the medially located tumours. In addition, several studies have pointed out that due to the large FoV of the camera and the bulky collimators, it is difficult to position the camera close to the breast, and thus, imaging breast tissue adjacent to the chest wall may not be possible. This may, ultimately, decrease the spatial resolution of the camera imaging system and thus affect the diagnostic value of the test in detecting such a small lesion size.

To overcome some of the limitations offered by conventional gamma camera on breast imaging, Gupta and colleagues [42] reported the first preliminary clinical data that are performed with breast-specific detectors and then compare it with the data obtained from standard full-size camera. A limited number of patients were investigated in this study but interestingly reported a higher sensitivity for the dedicated camera. Following this and due to the large research activities, new generation of detectors has been designed and developed for breast tumour imaging, for instance, the position-sensitive photo-multiplier tubes (PSPMT), semiconductor arrays and scintillation crystals coupled to an array of solid-state photo detectors.

The commercially available dedicated breast camera has two detectors and is designed and optimized to image only the breasts. It possesses a high intrinsic spatial resolution, and the camera is also equipped with ultra-high-resolution parallel-hole collimator and thus optimized for high-resolution SM. The main advantage of such cameras is the ability to separate the breast from the chest wall by positioning the camera close to the breast. Thus, the camera can be used in areas with limited space (e.g. medial view can be possible), where the use of a full-sized camera is impractical or impossible. The use of moderate breast compression capabilities may improve both the signal-to-nose ratio (SNR) and the spatial resolution [43] and thus increase the sensitivity for detecting smaller lesions. The proposed clinical indications for such dedicated cameras are similar to the full-size clinical gamma camera SM. There are some recent clinical studies associated with using these dedicated gamma cameras. For instance, a clinical preliminary study by Brem et al. [44, 45] using dedicated breast camera demonstrated a slight improvement in resolution and tumour sensitivity particularly for lesions~ 1 cm. Rhodes and colleagues reported [46] on SM performed on 40 women with small mammographic abnormalities (<2 cm) scheduled to undergo biopsy. The SM examination identified (33/36) malignant lesions confirmed at biopsy. The authors concluded that this preliminary study suggested an important role for the dedicated SM camera in women with dense breasts. In another study Brem and colleagues [47] evaluated 94 women (median age 55 years) presented with normal mammographic and physical examination results but all considered at high risk of developing breast cancer. Of these women 35 had a history of previous breast carcinoma or atypical ductal hyperplasia. The authors concluded that with this camera, they can depict small (8–9 mm) non-palpable lesions in women at high risk of breast cancer.

In summary, whilst these studies using breast-specific cameras are promising, all are considered preliminary in nature because they based on very few cases. Additional studies with a larger sample size are needed to accurately assess and reach scientific conclusions concerning these proposed cameras. They also need to be cost competitive with the general-purpose gamma cameras in order to be widely used in breast tumour imaging applications. In addition, the smallest lesion sizes that can be detected with these cameras claimed to be 3–3.3 mm [48] compared to 4–5 mm [49] with conventional camera. However, the evidence published to date did not demonstrate a statistically significant difference in lesion detection. The spatial resolution of these proposed cameras may further improve by increasing the pixel size, but there are however practical limitations in the development of cameras with small pixel sizes, including cost and detector design. More importantly due to the use of collimator, these dedicated cameras suffer from low detection efficiency. Nowadays, the latest revolution in the mammography field was announced by Dr. Jeffrey Shuren, director of the FDA's Center for Devices and Radiological Health, said on Friday, February 11, 2011 "Physicians can now access this unique and innovative 3-D technology that could significantly enhance existing diagnosis and treatment approaches". In addition, the US Food and Drug Administration approved on Friday the first X-ray mammography device that provides three-dimensional images of the breast for cancer screening and diagnosis.

3.1. Image reconstruction techniques

Screening and diagnostic mammography suffers from the limitation that the complex 3D breast structure is projected into a plane. Thus, lesions can be obscured by overlaying and underlying tissue structures which could cause a false negative, or dense overlapping tissue can mimic lesions, leading to an unnecessary recall of a patient. The proposed solution is 3D breast tumour image reconstruction techniques such as digital breast tomosynthesis (DBT) which is an emerging modality that produces 3D breast images. In DBT, lesion conspicuity is improved, which could potentially lead to earlier cancer detection and a more accurate diagnosis. In tomosynthesis, a volume image is created from a sequence of projection views acquired over a limited arc. Reconstruction from this data is challenging because the data is inherently incomplete. One-shot algorithms such as filtered back projection (FBP) have been developed for DBT image reconstruction. Though efficient, they tend to yield conspicuous artefacts. Iterative algorithms such as expectation maximization (EM) have also been employed with DBT. Such algorithms sacrifice efficiency but yield images with fewer artefacts. An additional drawback for EM, however, is that in general some form of regularization is needed which tends to reduce resolving power necessary for calcification detection.

3.2. Design details and preliminary results

3.2.1. Design details

The experimental system consists of a general radiography tube pointing at a given distance from the central axis of the breast. Four flat-panel digital detectors will be used to collect all the photon information (energy, flux, position) scattered by the phantom breast covering all possible area around it. The patient would lie on a table in the prone position with one breast drawn downwards through an opening to allow the X-ray tube and detector flat panels to be safely placed beneath the table (**Figure 1**).

During one irradiation of such phantom, we will investigate all the collected data to reconstruct the image in a 3D framework.

3.2.2. Preliminary results

As an illustrative example to indicate whether the proposed idea will work, we simulated a semi-spherical breast phantom including two air-filled cavities, irradiated with 10^8 photons. The photon energies imitate the standard spectrum of the commonly used X-ray source in mammography case studies. Monte Carlo sampling of the X-ray generator (30 kVp, Mo anode, filter 0.03 mm Mo and 1 mm Be) was carried out using the inverse cumulative method

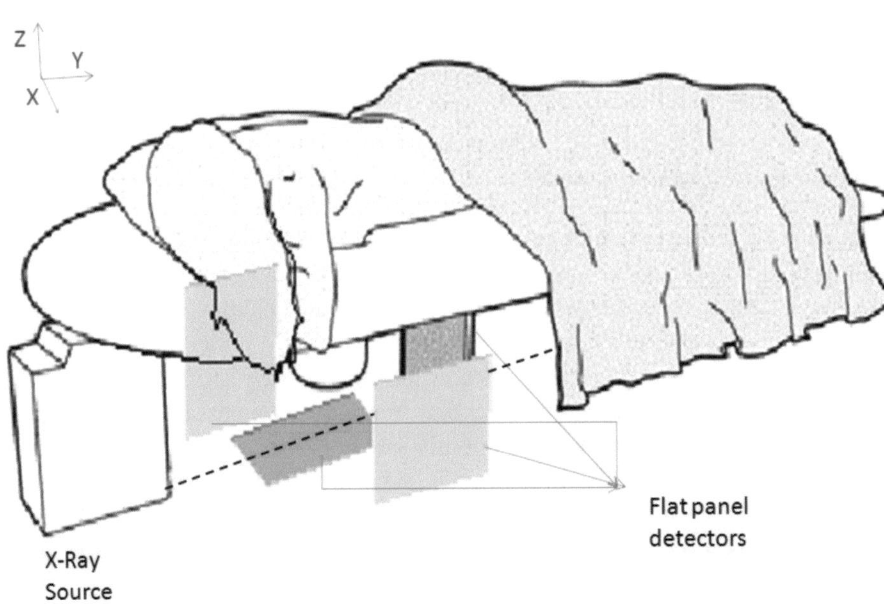

Figure 1. Schematic view of proposed setup design. Patient lies prone with one breast drawn downwards through opening in scanning device.

starting from experimental data sets. **Figure 2** shows the phantom (magenta colour) including two cavities (yellow) and surrounded with four flat-panel detectors (white). The two other faces contain the chest and the source beam zone.

The important data given by the scorers (flat-panel detector) numbers 2, 3 and 4 will contribute significantly on the final 3D image reconstruction process. **Figure 3** demonstrates how important the scattered photon statistics are for the given simulated setup.

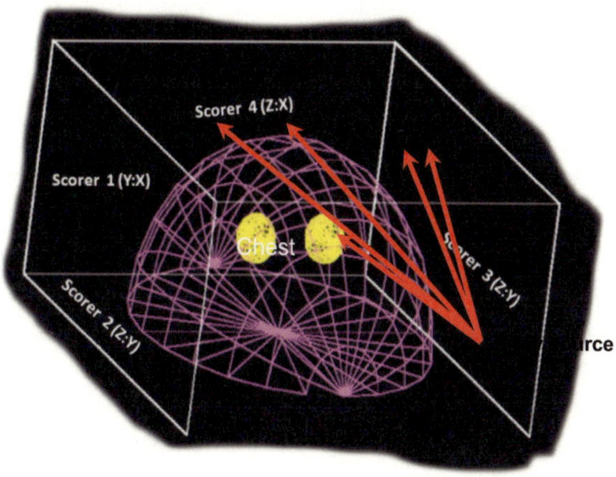

Figure 2. Simulated setup including the breast phantom (magenta), air cavities (yellow), X-ray photon (red) and the four scorers.

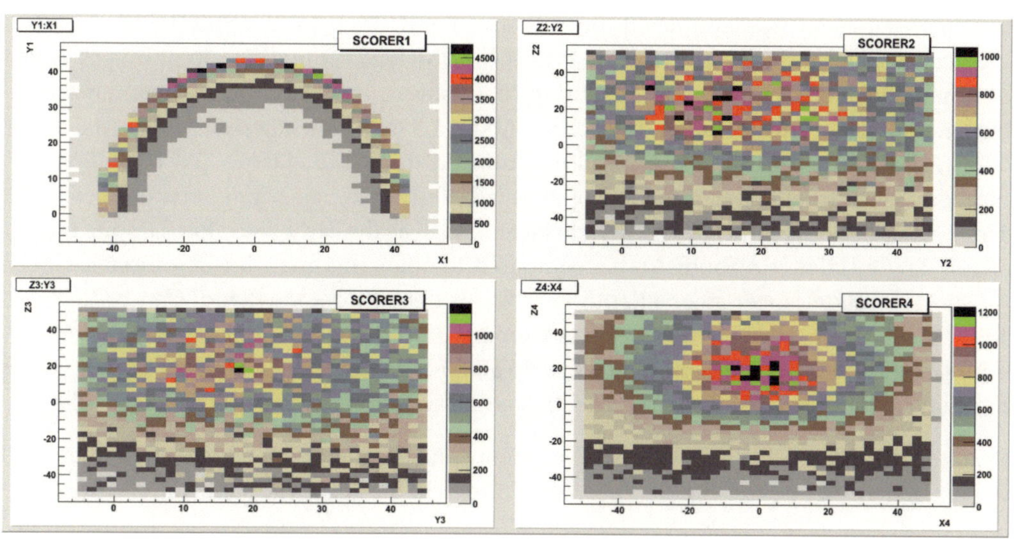

Figure 3. Simulated deposited energy using Geant4 Monte Carlo simulation toolkit for the four scorers. Bar scale indicates the specific magnitude of deposition.

Therefore, the goal of this project is to overcome all of the above limitations by providing a proof of concept for painless 3D mammography to be used as a screening and as diagnostic methods after commercialization. The proposed prototype includes (1) the detection system, which will be a set of semi-conductor arrays spatially distributed around each breast; (2) the X-Ray source; and (3) the convenient patients' test bed for painless exposition to X-rays. For that purpose, the first phase of the proposed project will focus on a versatile and widely used Monte Carlo simulation tool, Geant4, to optimize the detector arrays' chemical composition (CdZnTe, GaAs, etc.), spatial positioning around patient, source characterization (energy, spatial localization) and also the test-bed geometry to mainly fulfil the two conditions of radiation protection and painless positioning.

Secondly, we will use an iterative reconstruction algorithm to reconstruct the images of a mathematically breast phantom using the cluster network technique. Then, the experimental construction of the overall design will be carried out. Finally, the use of anthropomorphic breast phantoms to check the effectiveness prediction of the simulation will resume the project phases. Since most imaging modalities required a wide spectrum of capabilities which span biomedical sciences and physical sciences and clinical medicine, thus this project will be a collaborative cross-disciplinary research engaging together with scientist in universities and clinician in hospitals. Consequently, this proposal has the potential to score some successes in clinical imaging science. The project outputs will include the creation of a numerical platform able to more understand the breast disease problems and the development of an innovative prototype for painless breast imaging within a 3D framework. These allow the large communities of researchers and doctors to improve the breast imaging process and to build and to share some knowledge and experiences within that context. As a result, some international and national publications will be submitted to well-recognized journals.

Based on the assessment of current prevalence and projected incidence of diseases, cancer has been selected as medical and health-priority area for strategic intervention by the National Medical and Health Research Strategic Priorities (NMHRS) for the Kingdom. It is classified as a non-communicable disease [1]. Within that context, breast cancer is the second leading cause of cancer deaths in women today. About 1.3 million women are diagnosed annually worldwide, and about 465,000 will die from the disease. Incidence and mortality have reached a plateau and appear to be dropping in both United States and parts of Europe [1]. This decline has been attributed to several factors, such as the early detection. Despite the relatively low incidence in Saudi Arabia compared to other countries, breast cancer has been the most common cancer among Saudi females for the past decade (Saudi Cancer Registry, 1994–2005). The most concerned patients were aged between 40 and 50 years old. For that, a breast cancer screening programme will help all the female population, including the young one (having dense breast), for early detection and prevention advices.

So, the potential positive impacts on the economy and society of the current project are well defined in terms of decreasing the enormous burden to the healthcare-utilization costs.

Furthermore, the expertise to be developed through this project will be applied to the review of new digital radiographic imaging systems, the development of amendments to the diagnostic X-ray performance standard, the development of an advisory pertaining to national public breast cancer screening programmes and the joint planning of a consensus development conference on the 3D X-ray imaging modality with the King Saud University.

Also, investigating the computer-assisted diagnosis devices will provide the Kingdom with the scientific basis to effectively regulate this fast-growing field. In addition, this project may provide powerful tools of a commercial value for X-ray imaging application, especially with the development of such prototype, including the detectors, the source and the patient bed, that will meet to a 3D painless mammography.

Another benefit of such project concerns the supervision of two master's students and to create a locally competent talent capable of conducting novel medical and health sciences research. The creation of an infrastructure that supports and enables further research, in such medical field, will be an extra added benefit to the College of Applied Medical Sciences and to the King Saud University. The development and the setup of cooperative agreement by establishing collaborative research with advanced institutions such as the CERN and the University of Surrey will contribute to the technological opportunities transferred from over the world. Finally, the proposed project should participate in increasing national scientific discovery and productivity through promotion by publishing in peer-reviewed and reputable journals.

4. Valuable to the Kingdom

Based on the assessment of current prevalence and projected incidence of diseases, cancer has been selected as medical and health-priority area for strategic intervention by the National Medical and Health Research Strategic Priorities (NMHRS) for the Kingdom. It is classified as a non-communicable disease [1]. Within that context, breast cancer is the second leading cause of cancer deaths in women today. About 1.3 million women are diagnosed annually worldwide, and about 465,000 will die from the disease. Incidence and mortality have reached a plateau and appear to be dropping in both United States and parts of Europe [1]. This decline has been attributed to several factors, such as the early detection. Despite the relatively low incidence in Saudi Arabia compared to other countries, breast cancer has been the most common cancer among Saudi females for the past decade (Saudi Cancer Registry, 1994–2005). The most concerned patients were aged between 40 and 50 years old. For that, a breast cancer screening programme will help all the female population, including the young one (having dense breast), for early detection and prevention advices. So, the potential positive impacts on the economy and society of the current project are well defined in terms of decreasing the enormous burden to the healthcare-utilization costs.

Furthermore, the expertise to be developed through this project will be applied to the review of new digital radiographic imaging systems, the development of amendments to the diagnostic X-ray performance standard, the development of an advisory pertaining to national public breast cancer screening programmes and the joint planning of a consensus development conference on the 3D X-ray imaging modality with the King Saud University. Also, investigating the computer-assisted diagnosis devices will provide the Kingdom with the scientific basis to effectively regulate this fast-growing field.

In addition, this project may provide powerful tools of a commercial value for X-ray imaging application, especially with the development of such prototype, including the detectors, the source and the patient bed, that will meet to a 3D painless mammography.

Another benefit of such project concerns the supervision of two master's students and to create a locally competent talent capable of conducting novel medical and health sciences research. The creation of an infrastructure that supports and enables further research, in such medical field, will be an extra added benefit to the College of Applied Medical Sciences and to the King Saud University. The development and the setup of cooperative agreement by establishing collaborative research with advanced institutions such as the CERN and the University of Surrey will contribute to the technological opportunities transfer from over the world. Finally, the proposed project should participate in increasing national scientific discovery and productivity through promotion by publishing in peer-reviewed and reputable journals.

Author details

Mohammed Ali Alnafea

Address all correspondence to: alnafea@ksu.edu.sa

Department of Radiological Sciences, College of Applied Medical Sciences, King Saud University, Riyadh, Saudi Arabia

References

[1] King Abdulaziz City for Science and Technology. Strategic Priorities for Advanced Medical and Health Research, Doc. No. 39P0001-PLN-0001-ER01

[2] Apostolakis J, et al. GEANT – Detector Description and Simulation Tool, CERN Program Library Long Writeup W5013. Geneva, Switzerland: CERN; 1993

[3] Nelson WR, Rogers DW. Structure and operation of the EGS4 code system. In: Jenkins TM, Nelson WR, Rindi A, editors, Monte Carlo Transport of Electrons and Photons. New York: Plenum Press; 1988, pp. 287-305

[4] Briesmeister J. MCNP—A general Monte Carlo N-Particles Transport Code, LA 1265-M, Version 4B. Los Alamos, New Mexico, USA: Los Alamos National Laboratory; 1997

[5] Agostinelli S, et al. GEANT4—a simulation toolkit. Nuclear Instruments and Methods A. 2003;506:250-303

[6] Harris JR, Lippman ME, Verone U, Willett W. Breast cancer. New England Journal of Medicine. 1992;327:319-328

[7] The American Cancer Society. Cancer Facts and Figures 2006. Available from: http://www.cancer.org, retrieved on September; 2006

[8] Cavalli F, Hansen HH, Kaye SB. Textbook of Medical Oncology. Martin Dunits Ltd; 1998. ISBN: 1853172901

[9] Kelsey JL, Gammon MD. The epidemiology of breast cancer. Cancer. 1991;41:146-165

[10] Department of Health and Social Security, D. o. H. a. S., Ed., Breast Cancer Screening: Report of a Working group chaired by Professor Sir Patrick Forrest. London, UK: H. M. S. O; 1986

[11] Dufy SW, Tabr L, Chen HH, Holmqvist M, Yen MF, Abdsalah S, Epstein B, Frodis E, Ljungberg E, Hedborg-Melander C, Sundbom A, Tholin M, Wiege M, Kerlund A, Wu HM, Tung TS, Chiu YH, Chiu CP, Huang CC, Smith RA, Rosn M, Stenbeck M, Holmberg L. The impact of organized mammography service screening on breast carcinoma mortality in seven Swedish counties. Cancer. 2002;95:458-496

[12] Gøtzsche PC, Nielsen M. Screening for breast cancer with mammography. Cochrane Database of Systematic Reviews. 2009(4). Art. No.: CD001877. DOI: 10.1002/14651858.CD001877.pub3

[13] Kacl GM, Liu PF, Debatin JF, Garzoli E, Cadu RF, Krestin GP. Detection of breast cancer with conventional mammography and contrast-enhanced MR imaging. European Radiology. 1998;8(2):194-200

[14] Kopans DB. The positive predictive value of mammography. American Journal of Roentgen. 1992;158:521-526

[15] Hendee WR. History and status of X-ray mammography. Health Physics. 1995; 69(5)636-648

[16] Sankararaman S, Karellas A, Vedanthan S. Physical characteristics of a full-field digital mammography system. Nuclear Instruments and Methods in Physics Research A. 2004;533(14):560-570

[17] James JJ. The current status of digital mammography (Review). Clinical Radiology. 2004;59:1-10

[18] Adler DD, Wahl RL. New methods for imaging the breast: Techniques, findings, and potential. American Journal of Roentgenology. 1995;164:19-30

[19] Stefanoyiannis AP, Costaridou L, Skiadopoulos S, Panayiotakis G. A digital equalisation technique improving visualisation of dense mammary gland and breast periphery in mammography. European Journal of Radiology. 2003;45:139-149

[20] Pani R, Scopinaro F, Pellegrini R, Soluri A, Weinberg IN, De Vincentis G. The role of Compton background and breast compression on cancer detection in scintimammography. Anticancer Research. 1997;17(3B):1645-1649

[21] Alnafea MA, Wells K, Spyrou NM, Saripan MI, Guy M, Hinton P. Preliminary results from a Monte Carlo study of breast tumour imaging with low energy high-resolution collimator and a modified uniformly-redundant array-coded aperture. Nuclear Instrument and Method A. 2006;563:146-149

[22] Alnafea MA, Wells K, Spyrou NM, Guy M. Preliminary Monte Carlo study of coded aperture imaging with a CZT gamma camera system for scintimammography. Nuclear Instrument and Method A. 2007;573:122-125

[23] Kopans DB. The positive predictive value of mammography. American Journal of Roentgen. 1992;158:521-526

[24] Stavrous AT, Thickman D, Rapp CL, Dennis MA, Parker SH, Sisney GA. Solid breast nodule: Use of sonography to distinguish between benign and malignant lesions. Radiology. 1995;196:123-134

[25] Weinreb JC, Newstead G. MR imaging of the breast. Radiology. 1995;196:593-610

[26] Rankin SC. MRI of the breast. British Journal of Radiology. 2000;73(872):806-818

[27] Sharp PF, Gemmell HG, Smith FW. Practical Nuclear Medicine. USA: Oxford University Press. ISBN: 0-19-26284-0, 1-12; 1998

[28] Wahl RL. Current status of PET in breast cancer imaging, staging, and therapy. Seminars in Roentgenology. 2001;36(3)250-260

[29] Adler LP, Crowe JP, Alkaisi NK, Sunshine JL. Evaluation of breast masses and axillary lymph nodes with [F-18] 2-deoxy-2-uoro-D-glucose PET. Radiology. 1993;187(3):743-752

[30] Strauss LG, Conti PS. The application of PET in clinical oncology. Journal of Nuclear Medicine. 1991;32(4)632-648

[31] Strauss LG. PET in clinical oncology: Current role for diagnosis and therapy monitoring in oncology. The Oncologist. 1997;2:381-388

[32] Price P. Is there a future for PET in oncology? European Journal of Nuclear Medicine. 1997;24(6):587-589

[33] Bombardieri E, Aktolun C, Baum RP, Bishof-Delaloye A, Buscombe J, Chatal JF, Maoli L, Moncayo R, Mortelmans L, Reske SN. Breast scintigraphy: Procedure guidelines for tumour imaging. European Journal of Nuclear Medicine and Molecular Imaging. 2003;30(12):B107-B114

[34] Schillaci O, and Buscombe JR. Breast scintigraphy today: Indications and limitations. European Journal of Nuclear Medicine and Molecular Imaging. 2004;31:S35-S45

[35] Wiesenberger AG, Barbosa F, Green TD, Hoefer R, Keppel C, Kross B, Ma-jewski S, Popor V, Wojcik R, Wymer DC. A combined scintimammography/stereotactic core biopsy X-ray. Nuclear Science Symposium Conferece Record. 2000;3

[36] Fondrinier E, Muratet JP, Anglade E, Fauvet R, Breger V, Lorimier G, Jallet P. Clinical experience with 99mTc-MIBI scintimammography in patients with breast microcalci cations. Breast. 2004;13(4):316-320

[37] Schillaci O, Scopinaro F, Spanu A, Donnetti M, Danieli R, Di Luzio E, Madeddu G, David V. Detection of axillary lymph node metastases in breast cancer with 99mTc tetrofosmin scintigraphy. International Journal of Oncology. 2002;20(3):483-487

[38] Imbriaco M, Del Vecchio S, Riccardi A, Pace L, Di Salle F, Di Gennaro F, Salvatore M, Sodano A. Scintimammography with 99mTc-MIBI versus dynamic MRI for non-invasive characterization of breast masses. European Journal of Nuclear Medicine and Molecular Imaging. 2001;28(1)

[39] Buscome JR, Cwikla JB, Holloway B, Hilson AJW. Prediction of the usefulness of combined mammography and scintimammography in suspected primary breast cancer using ROC curves. Journal of Nuclear Medicine. 2001;42;3-8

[40] Fahey FH, Grow KL, Webber RL, Harkness BA, Harkness BA, Bayram E, Hemler PF. Emission tuned-aperture computed tomography: A novel approach to scintimammography. Journal of Nuclear Medicine. 2001;42(7):1121-1127

[41] Scopinaro F, Ierardi M, Porri LM, Tiberio NS, De Vincentis G, Mezi S, Cannas P, Gigliotti T, Marzetti L. 99mTc-MIBI prone scintimammography in patients with high and intermediate risk mammography. Anticancer Research. 1997;17:1635-1638

[42] Gupta P, Waxman A, Nguyen K, Phillips E, Yadagar J, Silberman A, Memsic L. Correlation of 99mTc-sestamibi uptake with histopathologic characteristics in patients with benign breast diseases [Abstract]. Journal of Nuclear Medicine. 1996;37(5):1122-1122

[43] Coover LR, Caravaglia G, Kunh P. Scintimammography with dedicated breast camera detects and localizes occult carcinoma. Journal of Nuclear Medicine. 2004;45(4):553-558

[44] Brem RF, Schoonjans JM, Kieper DA, Majewski S, Goodman S, Civelek C. High-resolution scintimammography: A pilot study. Journal of Nuclear Medicine. 2002;43:909-915

[45] Brem RF, Kieper DA, Rapelysea JA, Majewski S. Evaluation of a high-resolution, breast-specific, small-field-of-view gamma camera for the detection of breast cancer. Nuclear Instruments and Methods in Physics Research Section A. 2003;497(1):39-45

[46] Rhodes DJ, O'Connor MK, Phillips SW, Smith RL, Collins DA. Molecular breast imaging: A new technique using 99mTc-scintimammography to detect small tumours of the breast. Mayo Clinic Proceedings. 2005;80:24-30

[47] Brem RF, Rapelyea JA, Zisman G, Mohtashemi K, Raub J, Teal CB, Majewski S, Welch BL. Occult breast cancer: Scintimammography with high-resolution breast-specific gamma camera in women at high risk for breast cancer. Radiology. 2005;237(1):274-280

[48] Scopinaro F, Pani R, De Vincentis G, Soluri A, Pellegrini R, Porfri LM. High-resolution scintimammography improves the accuracy of technetium-99m methoxy-isobutylisonitrile scintimammography: Use of a new dedicated gamma camera. European Journal of Nuclear Medicine and Molecular Imaging. 1999;40:1279-1288

[49] Taillefer R. The role of 99mTc-sestamibi and other conventional radiopharmaceuticals in breast cancer diagnosis. Seminars in Nuclear Medicine. 1999;XXIX(1):16-40